praise for
good food, bad diet

"Abby Langer's new book has a simple but much-needed message: ditch the diet culture. Hear, hear! **This highly readable book maps a hype-free path to a realistic, sustainable, and healthy relationship with food and eating.** Along the way—with clarity and humor—Langer takes on celebrity culture, the diet and wellness industries, and our society's wayward obsession with youth and thinness. **A timely, fun, and science-informed read!**"

Timothy Caulfield, bestselling author of
The Science of Celebrity

"**Abby's no-nonsense approach to eating is a breath of fresh air in the sea of diet books.** If you've had enough of diet culture and categorization of food as 'good' or 'bad,' give this book a read. It will open your eyes to a realistic and doable approach to eating, while helping you accept your body and enjoy the food you consume to nourish it."

Toby Amidor, MS, RD, CDN, FAND,
award-winning nutrition expert and
Wall Street Journal **bestselling author of**
The Healthy Meal Prep Cookbook **and**
The Best 3-Ingredient Cookbook

"In a world overflowing with nutritional nonsense, **Abby Langer is the rare expert bringing light to dietary darkness.** *Good Food, Bad Diet* is exceptional."

James Fell, author of *The Holy Sh*t Moment*

"If diet culture has you so confused that you're not even sure what healthy eating looks like anymore, this is the book for you. *Good Food, Bad Diet* is **a total reeducation in nutrition**, one that will help you sort fact from internet fiction. Abby calls BS where she sees it and will guide you compassionately towards a healthier, happier you."

Desiree Nielsen, bestselling author of *Eat More Plants*

"In the wellness world of extremes, Abby offers a much-needed middle ground for those looking to improve their health without the physical and psychological risks of restrictive diets. *Good Food, Bad Diet* is **evidence-based, witty, and packed with accessible tips for anyone looking to live their healthiest, happiest life.**"

Abbey Sharp, RD, founder of Abbey's Kitchen

good food, bad diet

The Habits You Need to **Ditch Diet Culture**, **Lose Weight**, and **Fix Your Relationship** with Food Forever

abby langer, RD

published by simon & schuster

new york   london   toronto   sydney   new delhi

SIMON &
SCHUSTER
CANADA

Simon & Schuster Canada
A Division of Simon & Schuster, Inc.
166 King Street East, Suite 300
Toronto, Ontario M5A 1J3

This Simon & Schuster Canada edition January 2021

SIMON & SCHUSTER CANADA and colophon
are trademarks of Simon & Schuster, Inc.

For information about special discounts for bulk purchases,
please contact Simon & Schuster Special Sales at
1-800-268-3216 or CustomerService@simonandschuster.ca.

Manufactured in the United States of America

1   3   5   7   9   10   8   6   4   2

Library and Archives Canada Cataloguing in Publication
Title: Good food, bad diet : the habits you need to ditch diet culture, lose weight, and fix your relationship with food forever / Abby Langer.
Names: Langer, Abby, author.
Description: Simon & Schuster Canada edition.
Identifiers: Canadiana (print) 20200248243 | Canadiana (ebook) 20200248316
| ISBN 9781982137502 (softcover) | ISBN 9781982137519 (ebook)
Subjects: LCSH: Nutrition—Popular works. | LCSH: Weight
loss—Popular works. | LCSH: Food habits.
Classification: LCC RA784 .L36 2021 | DDC 613.2—dc23

ISBN 978-1-9821-3750-2
ISBN 978-1-9821-3751-9 (ebook)

contents

introduction:
good food, bad diet

Eating is the most primal instinct we have. We might not think about this fact day to day, but we need to eat to stay alive. In psychologist Abraham Maslow's Hierarchy of Needs, food is pretty much the highest priority, along with warmth and sleep. While it isn't required to find pleasure and emotional nourishment in food, that doesn't mean we should miss out on those aspects. Remember that moment as a kid when you bit into a sun-warmed, perfectly ripe peach? Or when you tried your first homemade chocolate chip cookie? It was incredible, right? And why shouldn't eating be incredible? Food has been bringing us together, not just for nourishment, but for pleasure and social connection, since the dawn of time.

Today, as then, having enough to eat is a privilege and something we can all be grateful for. And yet, in North America, where there is so much abundance, there are conflicting messages about what we should eat and what our bodies should look like—or not look like. This is called diet culture, and it has a chokehold on our society. It's made us physically and emotionally exhausted while simultaneously destroying what should be a fun and pleasurable experience.

Ever notice how many diets persuade us to shun foods that are "toxic" and "bad" in favor of "clean" and "good"? We label any sort of ultraprocessed food as bad, but why? You probably don't want to base your entire diet on them, but dirty? Nope. Food is not laundry. It's not "clean" or "dirty." To assign it those words is to condemn the nourishment that sustains our lives. It also deems those who make the "wrong" food choices as lesser, which is elitist and morally wrong. Intellectually, most of us know that someone who prefers Cheetos to a ten-dollar bag of kale chips is not "unclean" or "bad." But emotionally, many of us tend to believe the opposite because this is what diet culture has taught us. Person who eats Cheetos: bad, lazy, and unhealthy. Person who eats expensive kale chips: good, clean, and healthy.

Even seemingly harmless colloquial terms that are sometimes used to describe food, such as "guilty pleasure," "sinful," "cheat day," "naughty," and "guilt-free," have a destructive, underhanded meaning that categorizes anyone who eats as either devils or angels. This language hijacks the pleasure associated with food, and eating turns it into an anxiety-ridden moral dilemma: one that keeps plenty of us on the diet hamster wheel, going back and forth between good and bad, on and off the latest diet.

News flash: What you eat doesn't make you a good or bad person. Despite what our culture will have you believe, there is no association whatsoever with your diet and who you are. Using judgmental and moralistic terms to describe what we eat can create feelings of guilt and shame around food. If we overeat, we're weak. If we punish ourselves with diets, we're "being good." These labels are like little parasites that crawl into our brains and set up shop, subconsciously changing the way we feel about ourselves as people and influencing the choices we make in our food.

As food writer Bee Wilson states, "The moralising language around food encourages us to eat in ways that are both less plea- surable and also actually less healthy." We need to arrive at a space where eating certain foods is not a guilty pleasure, but instead is just plain pleasurable.

Let me tell you a story. Early in my career, I worked as a dieti- tian in a level-three trauma center. This hospital got the sickest, most mangled patients in their ICU, and I was the dietitian who looked after them. I saw a lot of bad stuff, but the cases that hit me the hardest were the people who were completely healthy one day, then suffered a catastrophic event like a car accident or a baseball bat to the head (truth) and were all of a sudden at the end of their lives. Many of these patients were younger than me and sometimes I had to leave the unit and go back to my office to take a moment to collect myself.

At the time, in my life outside the hospital, I spent a lot of time at the gym trying to burn off my dietary transgressions. I felt guilty about eating anything that didn't fit into my calorie allowance for the day and would cancel or decline plans to go for meals with people because I was afraid that I would overeat and gain weight. I felt immense pressure to look a certain way. Not because I was a dietitian, just because. I was miserable—physically exhausted from all the working out and emotionally exhausted from being so hy- pervigilant about everything I ate.

One day, as I stood at the foot of a hospital bed working on yet another tragic case, something occurred to me. This patient was a normal person yesterday. They had a job, friends, and a LIFE. Now they're never going to have those things again.

"So what am I doing?" I thought. "Are the few pounds I may or may not gain by enjoying my life worth all of what I'm giving up, socially, financially, emotionally?" If I was on my deathbed, would I be thinking, "Thank goodness I'm thin!" Or, would I regret saying no to those margaritas with my good friends and passing up the once-a-year pumpkin pie that my mom makes just so I could maybe save myself 0.6 of a pound? I knew the answer.

Life is short, and you need to grab it by the balls and swing it around every single day. Doing that means nourishing and caring for yourself physically and emotionally. It doesn't involve dieting and being miserable about food or shitty rules about burning fat and not eating gluten because it's toxic. It means rejecting diets and that game of tug-of-war with your body. It means setting yourself free and living IN THE PRESENT. That's worth everything.

Which brings me to the book in your hands. I want you to find pleasure, community, happiness, and comfort in food. It is one of the ways we can enrich our lives. There's a social dimension to eating that anthropologists will tell you has existed since the beginning of time, and for good reason: Food brings us together. It's an opportunity to share, to gather, to bond. And when you're relaxed about eating, that dimension opens up to you. But we can only get there when we begin to let go of what society has told us about food and our bodies.

In the chapters that follow, we're going to learn the truth about diet culture. I'll teach you why diets don't work and how they can actually damage your health instead of improve it. I'll help you re-examine your relationship with food—the "whys" behind what we eat—and once we find your "whys," we're going to examine them, feel them, and look them straight in the eye. I firmly believe that this is a necessary exercise to complete before making any changes to your diet. If you don't know where your feelings about food and your body are coming from, how can you see if they're negatively impacting your life? And how can you change them for the better? That's another step in this process that we'll be taking.

Together, we'll learn how to recognize true hunger from visual or emotional hunger and cravings. You'll map out feasible goals, whether that's finding a comfortable weight or eating more nutritious foods. We'll break down the basics of food and drinks—carbs, proteins, and fats—and how they nourish our bodies. Then I'll outline how you can put everything together in what I call high-value eating. We'll talk about nutrition and our gut health and the lifestyle changes we can make to safeguard both. Along the way, I'll be busting myths and answering all your burning questions about food, diets, and our bodies.

Before we go any further, let me make one thing clear: This book is NOT a diet book. I will never put you on a diet. We won't be talking calorie levels or meal plans or weight goals or restriction or cutting out entire food groups or saying no to your mom's lasagna. Because if you did any of that to me, I'd walk away, too. Screw that, I'll eat anything my mom makes and I will never count anything, ever. This book is also not for someone who is struggling with an eating disorder. If that's you, put this down and speak to your doctor. This book is not a replacement for individualized professional advice.

If you're looking for a book that holds your hand and tells you specifically which vegetables and fruits you should and shouldn't buy or that you need ½ cup of X and 3 oz. of Y, this isn't the book for you. You'll need to make friends with the fact that I'm going to let you find your own way in this and not just give you generic instructions on what to eat. I'm going to help you on every step of the journey, but this time, you'll truly learn how to nourish your body physically and emotionally. The truth is, we don't eat individual ingredients; we eat food. And food that nourishes us is both nutritious and pleasurable—that's true satisfaction.

I'm here to set the record straight: *All food is good and all diets are bad*. Once we understand that, we can start to move forward to a healthier place. Are you with me?

Let's do this!

ditch the diet

Even if you're not familiar with the term "diet culture," I have no doubt that you're familiar with the signs and symptoms, and the punishment they entail. Diet culture is a set of beliefs and norms that permeate through society, playing on our emotions around food and convincing us that we need to transform our bodies into something more "acceptable"—and that if we don't, we're failures.

Here's an example. When Beyoncé steps on a scale in her YouTube video promoting her twenty-two-day diet, she says to the camera, "This is every woman's worst nightmare," referring to either her weight gain, stepping on the scale, or both. Beyoncé's comment and the crazy, restrictive twenty-two-day diet she subsequently puts herself on are the perfect illustration of what diet culture is all about: Being fat is the worst thing that can possibly happen to us. Our "worst nightmare." Thanks, Beyoncé, but no. Gaining weight shouldn't be anyone's nightmare.

Diet culture tells us that if we gain weight, we need to fix ourselves with a punishing, restrictive plan to shed the weight, no matter the cost, because being fat is unacceptable. Fat is bad. Gaining weight is wrong. Stepping on the scale is scary. Martyring ourselves by starving is a badge of honor. The focus is only on how our body looks physically, with the sole desired outcome being an "acceptable" number on the scale, whatever that even means.

So, we do it, again and again and again. We eliminate foods that are harmless and healthy, such as dairy, wheat, and fruit. We talk about nothing with our friends except for what diet we're following and how it's working (or not). We show our kids that Mommy can't eat toast for breakfast, because toast isn't "good for us," and we snap at our partners because we're so fucking hungry we could actually gnaw our arm off. We turn down dinner dates with friends and that once-yearly pretzel at the baseball game and we feel like shit for eating some of our own birthday cake. All in the name of being thin and conforming to what diet culture says we should be.

Diet culture wants us to believe that we can't trust ourselves when it comes to food, which creates the perfect environment for us to think that we need diets, restrictive eating plans (don't cheat!) with specific instructions that will keep our bodies under control. The illusion that diets control our urges is just that: an illusion. *In reality, willpower and control are no match for our innate drive to eat, especially when we are restricting food.*

Diet culture sells an illusion. It sets out to convince us that we will only find happiness, achieve wellness, or be deemed beautiful if we're thin and young. Don't fit the mold? If so, diet culture wants you to believe that means you won't be a success in any aspect of your life. In other words, diet culture promotes the false idea that the only way to be worthy is to be thin.

This illusion of diet culture is something I see every day in my practice and in the world. It affects not only our food choices, but how we perceive ourselves and others. We weaponize the word "fat" when it relates to bodies, making it into an insult, when in reality, it's just a descriptive word. Calling someone fat is horrific. But calling someone thin is a compliment. This is because diet culture grabs us when we're young and tells us that fatter equals lesser and thinner equals better. And we're scared like hell of being lesser, so we'll do just about anything to be—and stay—thin.

We become convinced that all of our problems will suddenly vaporize when we fit into a size four, and that's a very compelling belief for anyone struggling with their weight. There's just one problem with this: It's all fatphobic bullshit. But people buy into it. There are many, many people with bodies of all shapes and sizes who are healthy and fit. The belief that weight loss is the only option because if you're not thin, you're not worthy, is a symptom of diet culture.

But here's the honest truth: All body colors, shapes, and sizes are beautiful, and no matter what you weigh or who you are, YOU ARE WORTHY. And here's something else: If you're a bigger person, *you don't have to lose weight.* Not everyone who isn't a size 0 wants to lose weight, needs to lose weight, or should lose weight. And screw diet culture for assuming all of that, too.

The funny (not funny ha-ha, funny weird) thing about diet culture is that it also has infiltrated the way we see aging. I think we'd all agree that aging is a natural process, but for some reason, we are so fucking afraid to get old. And even more than that, we are so afraid to look old. Diet culture has moved the needle on what it means to look your age, and put it in a place that's crazy and unrealistic for most women.

The perfect example is Jennifer Lopez, who is over fifty. When she performed with Shakira at the Super Bowl in 2019, people couldn't stop talking about how amazing she looked. This is now the standard to which women are being held as they age. Jennifer Aniston is another example. Thin, toned, and with the collagen matrix of a sixteen-year-old. But these women aren't the norm. And while I am so glad that women over fifty are taking up their space in the world—space that they deserve to occupy and always have— these celebrities are also increasing the pressure on normal women to look a certain way as they age. Where women over fifty were previously and unacceptably "invisible," the expectations are now at the other end of the spectrum, which is equally unfair. Thanks, diet culture. You suck.

The one thing that I do wish all women had that these celebrities have, is confidence and pride in how we look. Women are so used to focusing on what we perceive to be wrong with our bodies that we rarely focus on what we love about them. It's as though it's more socially acceptable to sit around and bitch with our friends about how fat our thighs look than it is to celebrate how strong and beautiful we are. It's fucked up that we aren't comfortable with feeling proud about our bodies. We're more comfortable with berating them. This has got to change.

In my work as a dietitian and food writer, I see that something is really wrong about the way we treat our bodies and how confused we are about food. Over the years, I became attuned to the colossal problem our culture has with eating and with the psychological, physical, and emotional abuse so many of us are putting ourselves through because we believe in magic fixes.

I've known plenty of people who rejected eating as a pleasurable activity in favor of the view that "food is fuel." They felt shame for finding happiness in food. Sound familiar? They forced themselves to be regimented and strict about eating and felt proud of themselves when they achieved that. Even though they loved food, they tried their hardest to hate it, or at least be indifferent to it. That way, it wouldn't hurt as much when they turned down the things they loved to eat and ate only the things they thought they should.

They believed that eating the right foods and looking the right way would help them feel better about their life and about themselves.

Spoiler alert #1: It never worked for them.

Spoiler alert #2: It's not likely to work for you either.

Call it a clash of values. Society's idea of the right body and the right diet may not be congruent with your personal beliefs about your body or about food. And trying to fit the mold that other people have created for diets and bodies will result in a tug-of-war that can last a lifetime, if you don't let that rope go and live your own truth.

I'll show you.

CASE STUDY: THE CHRONIC DIETER

Let me introduce you to Lisa. Because so many of us have been negatively influenced by diet culture, there's a little bit of her in all of us. Think of Lisa as a kind of composite client—a little like you, a little like me, a little like all of us who've struggled with fad diets, weight loss, and an obsession with being thin. In my practice, I see women like Lisa every day.

Lisa's unhappy with her weight. Why? She had kids and gained weight, then life got busy with two little ones, which didn't leave her much time to work out. Lisa sits in front of me on the couch in my office.

"Abby, I'm frustrated as hell," she says. "I keep dieting, but I'm fat and nothing works. I feel like a failure."

"What diets have you tried?" I ask her.

"Well, I've tried Weight Watchers, Paleo, keto, intermittent fasting, keto plus intermittent fasting . . . oh, and some weird meal replacement shakes and supplements someone on my Facebook page was selling."

"I'm sorry to hear none of those worked for you, but I'm not terribly surprised," I say.

"I just don't know what to eat anymore. It's so confusing and contradictory. One day, it's fasting. Then it's don't eat carbs. Next it's don't eat beans. Or avoid milk. I just want to know what to do. That's why I'm here. But I have to tell you: I hate diets. I never want to diet again!"

As Lisa tells me more about her various regimens, she has trouble keeping all the rules straight. But even after saying she never wants to be on a diet again, she reverts to diet-speak several times in our session, saying things like "I was bad last week with my eating" and "I have no willpower, I'm so weak" and "I feel like such a pig."

These are all things I've heard thousands of times over the years. Not just from clients either: from friends, family, men, teenage girls, and even at one point in my life, from myself. Even though these words are so familiar, they still set off alarm bells in my head. If you could describe the negative impact of diet culture in phrases, these are them. Honestly, when someone starts berating themself because of what they've eaten or describes themself as a pig, it makes me feel really sad. Who the fuck says? You think you're a farm animal known for gluttony because you ate an extra piece of cake? Come on.

As I look at Lisa sitting in front of me, I see that she probably isn't what would be considered clinically overweight, but she is obsessed with the number on her scale. Like many people I've met, she's always either on a diet or off one. When she's off, she lets herself eat whatever she wants, always knowing that she is going to "repent for her sins" by going on another diet as soon as possible. It's feast or famine. The result? She's lost and regained the same twenty pounds over and over again for eight years.

Like most of my clients who are chronic dieters, her mood suffers when she doesn't eat or when she's upset about eating too much, which affects her relationships with her husband and children. Her compulsive dieting cripples her sense of self-worth. More than anything, she wants to learn how to eat normally and live her best life, but the diets out there don't teach that sort of stuff. She also wants to "transform" her body to a pre-baby one, right down to her skinny jeans and carefree attitude. Lisa's insecurities, like her aging, postpartum body and her life as a mom, are a real concern for her, as they are for many women.

"What you're feeling is normal, and all too common," I say. "Your body is changing, which can be weird and concerning, but you deserve to be content with your body, with the food you choose, and with eating in general."

"That's what I want. But how?"

"By changing your relationship with food. It shouldn't be a source of guilt and pain. By really understanding that food is supposed to nourish you and help you thrive. It's going to be a process, but we'll get there, step-by-step."

Over and over in my practice, I've worked with people like Lisa whose relationship to food was broken and their health and wellness—both physical and emotional—were very much at stake. My goal has always been to bust through the many mythologies around diet culture and help my clients learn to love food, live healthier, and be truly well—inside and out.

The first step is working through their perception of themselves and their body, and figuring out where those perceptions originated. We also do a lot of work around their feelings about food and eating: Often, narratives that we learn in childhood affect those feelings, and I show clients how to flip those narratives to serve them instead of hurt them. This is something we'll be doing in the next chapter.

THE TRUTH ABOUT WEIGHT LOSS

Let me clarify where I stand on intentional weight loss because there are groups who advocate for the end of diet culture—way to go! I totally agree—but some also believe that we should stop trying to lose weight because it harms us physically and emotionally and we'll just gain everything back anyhow. And that's where my beliefs diverge with theirs.

While diet culture sucks, I do believe that there's such a thing as healthy weight loss, but from behavioral change, *not* from dieting. In other words, intentional weight loss doesn't need to be intertwined with diets and diet culture, nor is our only choice for weight loss either antidiet or restrictive diet. You can reject diet culture and still lose weight in a healthy manner. Weight loss does not have to involve restriction or punishment, which harms your relationship with food and your body. I don't believe—and this is important—in shaming someone for wanting to lose weight if it's for the right reasons, not because diet culture tells them to.

My friend Yoni Freedhoff, obesity physician extraordinaire, just completed a study that showed that *people are more likely to lose weight and keep it off if they enjoy their eating habits*. I mean, that's pretty obvious, right? If you hate something, you're more likely to give up on it. Human nature, and all.

Restrictive diets aren't that effective in the long run; most research that puts subjects on diets reveals that weight loss is tough and often short-lived. Although research subjects may be highly motivated to lose weight (which is probably why they sign up for the study in the first place), most studies don't allow them personalized recommendations or a focus on food quality rather than calories. Researchers often put participants on very low-calorie or very low-carb plans and don't necessarily address the emotional components of a person's relationship with food, which goes back years and years. Instead, they get a prescribed diet and then check in every once in a while. Great for short-term weight loss, not at all great for long-term behavioral change.

Just because something is a challenge doesn't mean you should give up and not do it, if it's something you want. But long-term weight loss can be tough, most definitely, for good reason: Aside from going on restrictive diets that are impossible to stick to, research shows that a good part of our weight is genetically determined, like the color of our eyes. I mean, colored contacts exist, but other than that, it's impossible to override genetics to change your eye color. Why attempt to do it with our weight?

Doing a deep dive into your feelings around weight and yourself is important work that we all need to do. Maybe it's not your weight you need to fix, but your relationship with food and your body.

A COMFORTABLE WEIGHT

If your goal *is* weight loss, ending up at a weight that you're comfortable at is more important than a specific number on the scale. A *comfortable weight* doesn't mean starving yourself, killing yourself at the gym, or feeling like you need to restrict your calories. It doesn't mean that you turn everything you put into your mouth into a number, either calories or macros, and have a running tally of what you've eaten in your head. That's not comfortable. At. All.

We all have a comfortable weight. You might not like yours because diet culture has convinced you that it should be a size four or that your body should look like an eighteen-year-old's when you're forty-five. This is insane and completely unrealistic. Repeat after me: It's not worth it to starve myself and lose joy from my life in order to fit diet culture's definition of what I should look like. Take it from me—it's more important to live your best life than to be constantly pissed about not fitting into a size six.

So, be realistic with your expectations for your body. Don't set number goals, because you have no idea how your body will respond to changes you make to your diet and lifestyle. Don't try to be the weight you were when you were twenty-five, if you're several decades older than that. Weight gain as we age is normal. Release the vise grip that you have on a certain number or "look" for your body. If you feel like you need to lose weight, what you should be aiming for is a comfortable or happy weight that you can maintain without much effort. One that feels natural to you because it's simple to maintain with small changes that are easy.

The secret to maintaining a comfortable weight for the long-term is:

- ✕ Understanding that food and eating never play nice with guilt and shame.
- ✕ Fixing your relationship with food and your body by figuring out and resetting your negative core beliefs.
- ✕ Understanding how your body works and why food restriction backfires.
- ✕ Improving the quality of what you eat.
- ✕ Knowing the difference between a comfortable weight and a weight that's unrealistic.

✖ Adding, not taking away, foods that you enjoy eating.

✖ Customizing your eating so it feels natural to you.

✖ Doing some physical activity.

✖ Recognizing that some days you'll need more, some days you'll need less.

✖ Learning to recognize the diet bullshit you see online and pretty much everywhere, for what it is: bullshit.

In short, the path to achieving and maintaining a comfortable weight is understanding your relationship around food and eating, coupled with behavioral change, accurate information about food, and a solid understanding of how your body works. The goal of this book is to equip you with all that.

So, what if you think diet culture sucks, but you still feel like you're not at a comfortable weight for you? The desire to lose weight is not always influenced by diet culture, despite what some people believe. Some of you might be doing it for health reasons. Or, you've recently put on weight from less-than-ideal eating habits. That's okay.

But if you're a chronic dieter, always looking for a way to lose weight, chances are you're not just doing it because you just want to drop a few pounds. It's tough to find someone who continually punishes themself without an underlying reason, so if you have one, you're going to find out what it is (and neutralize it) in the coming chapters.

If you're wondering if you've been influenced by diet culture, here are some diet-related behaviors that you might recognize:

✖ You've felt the guilt of eating something "bad," like freshly baked cookies, or an ice cream on a hot day, even if it was with your kid, a friend, or your partner.

- You've skipped dinners with friends because you were afraid of breaking your diet.
- You've said no to your mom's fabulous freshly baked bread because you weren't eating carbs.
- After making sacrifices like the ones above, you've felt proud about how much self-control and discipline you have.
- When you go off your diet, you go wild. It starts with a "cheat day," or maybe a handful of chips or a donut in the lunchroom at work. The dam breaks, and you can't control the urge to eat. Everything. In. Sight. Overeating sometimes is normal, but what I'm talking about here is a loss of control followed by guilt and shame, which brings me to . . .
- You've felt guilty for failing to control your eating. And the guilt is so overwhelming that you decide to "be good" again and start restricting your food intake or calories. "This time it's going to be different," you tell yourself. "I'm going to do better."

Here's the thing: These thoughts and behaviors are very real, and they make you feel extremely shitty. They're symptoms of a culture that sells you a dream but will only lead you around and around the shame circle as you chase the myth of thinness.

And the worst part? Even if you lose weight because of your deprivation, it's a diet culture bait and switch: You'll still be the same person with the same problems. You'll just be thinner. Diet culture tells us that we'll be a different, happier person if we can push through and lose weight, but that's all bullshit. Submit to diet culture's charms, and you'll be miserable AF because your issues will still be there, plus you'll be starving and isolated.

When you become conscious of the harm diet culture causes, you can begin to embrace a new and healthier paradigm.

watch out:

for "wellness."

Once the concept of dieting was starting to overstay its welcome, the wellness industry moved right in to claim its space. How convenient! Weight Watchers became WW, claiming that its primary focus was shifting to "wellness." Goop was born (I rue the day). Wellness exploded into a $4.5 trillion industry with some beneficial offerings (employee wellness programs) and many scams (IV vitamin drips, celery juice, diet companies masquerading as wellness programs).[1]

The one consistent thing about the wellness industry is that it promotes the concept of thinness as the apex of health. This is completely false: A person can be thin and desperately unhealthy both physically and emotionally. In other words, more often than not, wellness is just another word for "diet."

Instead of being inclusive—because we would all agree that wellness in its purest form should be available to everyone on earth—it's disgustingly exclusive with its forty-dollar reformer classes and nine-dollar grass-fed butter that has no evidence to support using it over the regular stuff, thank you very much. Most wellness companies don't really care about you; they care about making money. #Truth.

And we can't talk about money and wellness without talking about wellness influencers. Hop onto Instagram, and you'll find #fitspo posts of impossibly thin people drinking green juice and spouting "inspirational" messages such as "sweat is fat crying." While they might look healthy, if you're following influencers for nutrition information, you're probably getting only half of the story—the other half being that many health influencers are not at all healthy emotionally or physically after subjecting themselves to extreme eating and exercise habits.

Having spent time in that world, I can corroborate that assertion. Social media is a cesspool of terrible nutrition and body messages.[2] Much of what you see posted by professional influencers on social media is curated, meaning it's fake. It's edited, shot, and reshot, one photo in a hundred that they chose because it's perfect. It's paid for, Photoshopped, and worst of all, it's a fairy tale meant to sell you something. It's not real life.

But that doesn't stop us from looking to social media influencers for nutrition and health information, even though very few give accurate information on those topics.[3] So, needless to say, if you're getting the majority of your facts on social media, you might want to reconsider your sources.

Let's not forget the impact that seeing the so-called perfect lives of influencers has on the rest of us: Research has shown that people who spend time on Instagram have a lower body image and are most at risk for anxiety, depression, and eating disorders.[4,5] Instagram influencers and food bloggers push "clean eating" in the guise of health, but let's face it: Long-term fasts and "cleanses" are unnecessary and are bound to cause rebound eating . . . which of course, we blame on ourselves and our lack of willpower.

If you're following people on social media who make you feel like shit about yourself or your diet, it's time to unfollow them. I promise you, you won't regret it.

For someone who is a chronic dieter and/or has fraught relationships with food and their body, making peace with eating can seem like an impossible goal. I know how it feels, because I've been there. I understand how terrifying it can be to imagine letting go of the "rules" to end up floating untethered in a world awash with donuts, chips, steak, and every type of food you've been told you shouldn't be eating. It involves breaking the habit of dieting and restricting food. It's like moving into a new universe where food and eating can be enjoyable and fun, not a source of shame. It's giving diet culture the finger and walking away. Those changes can be very scary and very daunting.

If you're a chronic dieter, this fear is your story. It has likely consumed years of your life and has had an exorbitant cost on your social, emotional, financial, and physical health. It has become an addiction of sorts, a habit you can't seem to break. Unfortunately, diet culture will always exist, but that doesn't mean it has to control you. It's time for you to be free.

In the chapters that follow, I'm going to teach you how to reexamine your relationship with food, let go of your diet forever, and embrace a whole new outlook on yourself, what you eat, and why.

So, ask yourself right now: "Am I ready to let go of my dieting behavior?"

Maybe your answer is yes, maybe it's a no. Either way, I'll be here to guide you. Ready for more? Keep reading.

find your core beliefs

The most important part of healing your relationship with food is recognizing the psychological issues you may have with eating. In the first chapter, we discussed diet culture and its negative influence. Now let's talk about how to set the stage for true change to happen.

The first step is looking within and understanding your psychological relationship with food and your body. A lot of books and experts won't touch this subject because it can be really messy and unpleasant, and it doesn't end in a set promised goal of pounds lost or the perfect "bikini body." But the truth is that chronic dieting and poor body image are symptoms of something deeper that needs to be hauled up and explored. *We aren't born hating our bodies.* That's a learned behavior. We learn to starve ourselves and hate what we see in the mirror. It's time to unlearn that shit because nobody deserves to live their life like that.

Being bound up by the past and by feelings you're not acknowledging can keep you from moving forward and living your best life. Although it can be tough to face what's really going on inside of you, only by unpacking the feelings and origins behind your eating behavior will you be able to take the next step toward wellness and make meaningful, lasting change to your diet and in your life. Remember: You want to live in the present and be present for your life and the people you love.

So, what's the secret? Understanding your core beliefs.

WHAT ARE CORE BELIEFS?

Core beliefs are internalized messages or truths that we hold very close to our hearts. They determine how we see ourselves in the world and how we perceive the world around us, and they shape our sense of self-worth and our life decisions. In other words, your core beliefs are pretty damn important to your emotional health, especially if you're trying to heal your relationship with food and your body.

Core beliefs start young. This is normal—we're not born with beliefs, we're taught them. As impressionable children, we believe anything and everything that's told to us or modeled for us by an authority figure.

Core beliefs can be positive. For example, if your grandfather told you that you were smart as a child, and if over time, this was reinforced and you came to believe it was true, that core belief would engage whenever you needed it. For instance, when you were anxious about an exam or a project, you might have tapped into your core belief to remind yourself that you were capable. It's like a pocket of confidence you carry around everywhere you go. Yay for positive core beliefs!

When it comes to our bodies, positive core beliefs are validating and inspiring. Even if the core beliefs are superficial like "I have beautiful skin" or "I have amazing stamina," they can go a long way in making us feel good about ourselves and giving us confidence. When faced with a new fad diet that is selling you vitamin supplements for better skin, you can always say, "Nah, I already have beautiful skin. No, thanks." We like positive core beliefs, but unfortunately, the everyday world of marketing wants to undermine them by selling us fear and negativity about ourselves.

So it will come as no surprise that core beliefs can also be negative—and the negative ones are so much stickier than the positives. If you grow up being told by a parent, relative, or someone you know (or don't know) that your body doesn't fit, that's it's too big, or that you're not good enough, you'll probably believe it eventually. Why? Remember what Julia Roberts said in *Pretty Woman*? "The bad stuff is easier to believe." She's right. *If someone—or even you—tells you something negative enough times, you're going to start taking it as the truth.* It's called negative bias, and you can blame evolution. In the Stone Age, if we heard about something bad happening, our brains would tune out other stuff in order to focus on getting us away from the perceived danger. Over time, we became more aware of negative things as preemptive measures against harm. Unfortunately, today we don't need negative bias as much to survive, but its remnants exist. Hence we believe bad things easily and they tend to overshadow the good.

It happens to everyone. If I get sixty compliments on social media and one shitty rude comment from some idiot, that rude one is the only one I focus on. Well, until I remember my own advice. But still, focusing more on the negative is totally normal.

If you're a chronic dieter (or even if you're not), you probably feel bad about some part of your body. You might habitually criticize yourself and your diet. The key word is "habitually." You might be doing all of this subconsciously many times a day, but what's actually happening is the manifestation of your negative core beliefs. They bubble up into the nasty things we tell ourselves about our bodies and about the foods we eat—it's like a movie reel on repeat. You can be the smartest, most accomplished person in the world and still have these horrible thoughts about yourself. Not only that, but negative core beliefs tend to keep us in the past, all wrapped up in beliefs that aren't necessarily even true, and unable to move forward with happiness and freedom in our bodies and in eating.

When we experience stress or change in our lives, our negative core beliefs can be triggered. For someone with negative core beliefs about themself, a trigger event such as weight gain, a week in which you feel as though your diet isn't the greatest, or a clothes shopping trip can revive those negative core beliefs that might have been lying dormant. You might start believing crap: that you're lesser because you can't fit into that bikini you want or that you're weak because you gained so much weight during your vacation.

If you think about these statements, you may realize—correctly, I should add—that they're completely untrue. But most of us don't take the time to reason with ourselves. Instead, we play our movie again and again in our mind: a repeat of those same shitty things about ourselves, to ourselves. If that reel is negative, it can chip away at your self-esteem and happiness. Many of us even bury these thoughts and let them occur subconsciously because it's a lot easier to let the movie play, underneath everything, unchallenged and unchecked.

You may not be entirely aware of just how many negative core beliefs are actually impacting your choices, thoughts, and behaviors around food. They may be why:

✄ You feel a compulsive need to go on diet after diet.

✄ You're never satisfied with how your body looks, moves, or fits.

✄ You berate yourself, playing your negative reel in your head and making disparaging comments about yourself to others.

✄ You constantly feel like you're chasing something—a body-shape illusion—that you just can't seem to catch.

✄ You're so exhausted with the effort of all of these things. Just so exhausted.

✄ You believe that because of what you weigh and what you eat, you deserve to be punished.

All of that is fucking bullshit.

You don't deserve any of that garbage. Your body is perfect the way it is, and it deserves to take up space. It deserves respect. After all, it's working hard to keep you alive and doing what you do, every day. Plus, it's uniquely yours. Stand up for it, because nobody else can. Nobody (and no body) in the world deserves to be punished for eating. I don't give a crap if you've eaten cake or vegetables, it's all GOOD. And you should be enjoying it.

We'll get to that, but first, we need to identify those negative core beliefs so we can oust them for good. They're trolls, just lying in wait, coiled up and ready to pounce. Calling out these little shits is the first step in eradicating them. Let's go.

DITCHING THE TROLLS

Negative core beliefs sell us the fallacy that we're broken in some way and will never be good enough, and this causes us to continually punish ourselves physically and emotionally in an attempt to repent for and fix what you think is wrong. It's like we're constantly trying to push a boulder up a hill and it continues to roll on top of us again and again. Not okay! Even if you reach your goal, be it weight loss or anything else, you might not find satisfaction and peace, because deep inside you still believe you're not good enough. There's that boulder again. Ouch.

Until you shine a light on your negative core beliefs, they will continue to roll on top of you and hold you back. The only way to address them is to expose them. Remember, other people don't get to define who you are. That's your job. So whatever ideas you've been handed about yourself need to be inspected. Sit with them and acknowledge them. This might be uncomfortable (and it probably will be) because our first instinct may be to hide those feelings away in a box and tape the lid shut. But hold steady. Keep that box open and you will truly see where your feelings are coming from. Only then can you disable the power of your negative core beliefs and keep the positive ones.

This process can be painful and can cause all kinds of emotions. Seriously, it can really suck. But it's a necessary exercise in order for you to move forward. And if you find this at all triggering, there's no harm (and often a lot of good!) that can come from talking with a qualified professional therapist. Don't be afraid to find someone who will walk with you through this and give you the support that you need.

In the exercise below, I've listed the five most common negative core beliefs people have around weight, food, and eating and illustrated them with examples from my practice. But before each scenario, I've asked some important questions that I want you to answer about your relationship with food and your body.

The intention here is to get you to think about your own core beliefs and then turn the negatives into positives. It's a three-step process: The first step is calling out what our negative core beliefs are. This takes their power away. It's like realizing that the person who has been trolling you online is actually not that scary in real life. Once you realize who they are, you're so much more able to ignore them and anything they say to you. The second step is challenging the belief, then flipping it into a positive. This will change that movie reel of yours into a story with good, encouraging messages . . . all day long.

Okay, let's get started.

Question #1: What were you taught about food and weight when you were growing up?

Can you remember any messages you received about your body and your weight when you were a child? Maybe it's that moment when your mom put you on a scale at eight years old and told you that you weighed too much. Or when those asshole kids at school bullied you for being different or bigger than everyone else. What did this tell you about food and weight? That your body wasn't good enough? That diets are a necessary way of life in order to conform and be accepted? That thin is perfect? Really think about your answer. Write it down if you want.

Core belief #1: Thin = lovable. Thin = attractive.

For many people, this core belief forms at an early age. But the first messages we receive about our bodies and food aren't always overtly communicated. For one client of mine, her parents modeled their beliefs for her: "My parents were always on a diet, and it made me feel like I had to measure up physically at all times. I mean, if they considered themselves to be fat, what did they think of me? I never wanted to find out. At fifty-six years old, I still feel that pressure, even though both my parents are in their nineties. Somewhere inside of me I feel like I'd still be a disappointment to them if I slip and gain weight."

This is called "transgenerational transmission," which means that the beliefs and rules and culture of the family come down through generations, and they can be really tough to shift. Even though it wasn't their intention, my client's parents reinforced the message that fat was unacceptable, that gaining weight was akin to being a bad person or a weak person. My client absorbed this, and as a result, she became a chronic dieter at a very young age in order to keep herself in her parents' good graces. Subconsciously, even well into adulthood, she felt as though she owed it to the family to conform and her diet mind-set became a negative core belief.

We don't even have to be subjected to continual negative talk about our bodies or diet in order to form a negative core belief. A one-off comment can turn into a little demon that we fixate on and allow to warp our relationship with food and ourselves for years to come. Like my client whose teacher made a rude, inappropriate, offhand comment about how she wouldn't be able to fit behind her desk at school. Now every time she sits at a desk or a seat on an airplane or in a movie theater, she's reminded of that remark. Even though in her rational mind as an adult she knew that the teacher's comment was about the teacher, not her, she still internalized her anger and it continued to prevent her from making meaningful changes to her lifestyle and eating habits.

Growing up in an environment where our natural cues are questioned, belittled, and suppressed can also have damaging results. One client's story always stands out for me: "I was on the swim team in high school, so I was always hungry. When I would reach for seconds at the dinner table, my mom would always make a comment about how I didn't need the extra food. I think I've always believed that she'd rather I starved than be fat. And that her love was obviously conditional on how I looked. I think that's why I've starved my own body for the past thirty years."

Here was an active and healthy young woman who was taught to question her natural hunger cues but also equate them with her worthiness to be loved. The message was very clear: "Your body is wrong. If you listen to it, you will become fat and unlovable." The truth is that our natural cues are what keep us alive and thriving in whatever environment we end up in. We're supposed to eat when we're hungry; it's a natural physiological reaction and suppressing that urge can be dangerous.

These stories encapsulate how experiences from our childhood can warp our mind-set and push us to create unhealthy narratives that we continue to replay in our minds. We walk through life telling ourselves, "I am unattractive unless I'm thin" and "I'm not lovable unless I look a certain way." It doesn't matter that we intellectually know that these statements are untrue. In the end, we create rules and expectations that are unrealistic and unhealthy, like being hypervigilant about our eating habits and our weight, chronic dieting, having a poor self-image, and feeling guilt and shame around eating.

For all of these clients, their negative core belief was that if they weren't thin, they were unlovable and unattractive. Does any of this resonate with your answer to question #1? If so, it's time for step two.

Question whether this core belief is true.

Ask yourself if you believe that your weight determines your worthiness. If the answer is yes, try to remember whose voice you hear telling you this untruth. Did this core belief actually come from you or is it somebody else's opinion that you've assumed for yourself? Ask this negative core belief for proof. What makes you believe that it is really true?

Now that we have that settled, on to step three.

Flip your negative core belief into a positive.

For example, you might say, "Everybody is inherently worthy of love and affection, regardless of how they look." Or, "Nobody gives a shit about how much I weigh. It's irrelevant to who I am as a person, a friend, a partner, and a parent."

Now prove that this new, positive core belief is true. For example, write down evidence of what makes you worthy of love and happiness. What do you do for others? Why do others love you? How do you support your kids, your friends? What do you contribute to people's lives? These can be things like being there for someone when they need you, or being aware of injustice in the community and trying to right it. Listing the evidence to back this up strengthens the belief and weakens the negative one so you can truly pitch it into the trash where it belongs. What are you finding?

Question #2: Do you consistently use food to cope with emotions, particularly negative ones?

If so, where did this come from? What do you eat during these moments? What impact do these eating behaviors have on your emotional state? Were you ever punished or rewarded with food, and how do you feel this has impacted you? This is a tough one. Take your time answering.

Core belief #2: Food = safety. Food = love.

Humans have a much more complex relationship with food than, say, animals, who only eat to survive. We enjoy an epic cake on a birthday, not because we are hungry, but because celebrating with food is fun. But the flip side is, we also use food to soothe, to manage our emotions, and even to reward ourselves.

I had a client who came to me for weight-loss counseling. At fifty-two years of age, he had a thing for orange Tang drink crystals and drank liters of Tang every day. "I can't stop drinking it," he said. "My dad used to give it to us kids when we were young, especially at celebrations and when we did something he was proud of. He died when I was eleven, but I still remember the happiness that came with that Tang." My client was self-aware enough to recognize the emotions driving him to drinks liters of this stuff. He was trying to recapture something that was gone—his father's love—and who could blame him? After experiencing loss at such a young age, he was doing anything he could to hold on to memories of his father.

Another client of mine grew up in a family in which her parents constantly fought and her sisters always got into fistfights. At seven years old, she didn't have the maturity or coping skills to deal with all this conflict, so when the fighting began, she'd grab a bag of chips and sequester herself in the attic. She was out of harm's way with yummy food, and she felt safe.

As an adult, she employed the exact same coping mechanism: Whenever she felt anxious or unsafe, she'd retreat to a quiet place with a bag of chips. Again, who could blame her? It worked when she was a child; why shouldn't it as an adult? But the consequences of this habit caught up with her. She gained a lot of weight and her health was beginning to suffer.

In both my clients' cases, there's a scientific reason for their behavior: serotonin. Affectionately called "the happy chemical," serotonin is a neurotransmitter that's mostly made in the gut. When we eat, especially large amounts of food, serotonin is released; it makes us feel full and lifts our mood. This would be great if everyone was eating salads and vegetables and getting a serotonin high. Unfortunately, studies have found a correlation between being upset and getting a high after reaching for "unhealthy foods" like carbohydrates, sugar, and anything we would deem junk food or comfort food. Over time, we associate these foods with safety and happiness and use them as a way to numb our emotions, especially when we face tough situations.

All of us engage in emotional eating at some point, which is completely normal and definitely nothing to worry about, as long as you have—and use—other coping mechanisms. Having your mother's chicken soup while you're sick or enjoying ice cream after a bad breakup makes us human. It's a complex relationship, but it pains me to see clients who use food to protect themselves and find safety from the situations that life sometimes throws at us. At the end of the day, food should help us feel nourished, energized, and ready to take on the world. It shouldn't be used repeatedly to help us feel safe and protected from the world. Which brings us to step two.

Question whether this core belief is true.

Do you believe your food replaces love? Do you believe you're not worthy of love from other sources? Does food make you safe? Do you have the power to get through the tough situations that pop up in life?

Flip your negative core belief into a positive.

For example, "Food is food, and it doesn't love me back. That's okay, though, because I sure as hell am loved by actual people. And food doesn't make me any safer. I'm capable of using other skills and supports to create a safe place for myself without food."

Why do you know that this new, positive core belief is true? Remember, articulating the reasons why will reinforce the belief. It might take some reminding, but you'll get there. In the meantime, know that you are loved and safe.

Question #3: Do you think you'll be a different or better person once you lose weight?

Do you believe that you're worthy of health and happiness? Ask yourself where this idea comes from. Don't be afraid to be honest with your answer. We're going beyond the superficial here.

Core belief #3: Thin = worthy. Thin = a better life.

Of all the core beliefs, this is a hard one to dismantle because we see it and experience it everywhere—influencers on social media, advertisements, and celebrities hawking fitness products keep telling us what a "normal" body should look like and that being thin is better. So I understand friends, family, and clients fantasizing about being thin because they see it as a way of becoming a better person and as a transformation for their lives. The problem is that it's just not true.

Dayna was a mom of four kids who came to me for weight-loss counseling. She had a history of trying to change her eating habits, but as she told me, she was "never able to keep it going." She told me that because of her kids' busy schedules, her husband's food preferences (he hated certain vegetables and fish, so she didn't make those things), and her own job demands, she just couldn't "stay on track." And in our sessions, she continually spoke about weight loss as though it would make everything in her life fall into place. If only.

What I was hearing was that Dayna always put herself last—everyone's wants and needs were more important than hers. The actor Teri Hatcher called this the "burnt toast syndrome." People, especially mothers, give everyone else the perfectly toasted pieces of bread, leaving the burned, less desirable pieces for themselves so as not to inconvenience anyone else. They don't believe they are worth the effort of making another, unburned piece of toast for themselves. Their core belief is that they're not worthy of health and happiness; they're not important but everyone around them is. Dayna felt guilty for putting her needs first, so she sabotaged her efforts to change her eating habits over and over again, and when she inevitably failed to achieve them, she felt even more unworthy.

Having damaged self-worth is an issue in a lot of respects, but in terms of eating and body image, it can have a serious impact. People whose core beliefs include worthlessness are more likely to suffer from eating disorders, speak harshly to themselves, punish themselves unnecessarily, and experience excessive guilt and shame, especially when they feel as though they've made a mistake.

I've had to work hard to convince clients like Dayna that accepting their own worth and putting themselves as a priority is the first step toward change. And beyond that, to convince them that weight loss or weight gain is only one part—a very small part—of their success story, that being thin is not going to make them a better mother or husband or help them get the corner office or a nicer car or their dream job. All losing weight does is change how we look. It doesn't heal a bad relationship with food or with your body, and it doesn't turn you into someone else. You'll still have most if not all of the same problems, the same life, the same family. You'll just be thinner. And being thinner doesn't automatically equip you to deal with life any better. You are more than just the sum of your parts.

For any meaningful change to occur in your life, you need to believe and understand you are worthy of that change. If you hold the negative core belief that you're not worthy because you're not thin, it will be tough to achieve or sustain any sort of behavior change that leads to weight loss because you'll be continually going back to the habits that support that negative belief. It's also important to acknowledge that if you lose weight, your life will still be mostly the same. Magical unicorns and a whole new, sparkling life aren't going to jump out from behind the bathroom wall when the scale finally reads that certain number. Many things in our lives can be changed, but weight loss won't do that work for us.

Question whether this core belief is true.

Do you believe that losing weight will make you a better person and more worthy of respect and love? Do you think weight loss will change your life? How and why? What evidence can you find?

Flip your negative core belief into a positive.

Tell yourself, "How I look has no bearing on who I am as a person. I'm worthy of all good things, regardless of what I weigh." Think about someone you know and love. Would you not like them as a person as much if they gained weight? You probably would never dream of doing that. So, why do you believe it to be true for yourself?

Now list the reasons that this new, positive core belief is true. What does this tell you?

Question #4: Do you trust yourself to make good food choices?

If not, why? Where did this come from? When you were younger, did you choose what you ate or did others? And to what degree? Examine your level of self-trust around food and evaluate the impact of this on your core beliefs. Now that you're an adult, who makes your food choices? Do you feel you have control over what you eat or does someone/something else? Interesting, right?

Core belief #4: I can't be trusted and neither can my body.

This is one of the more common issues my clients have, and it often stems from the negative core belief that there is something wrong with their moral compass or their body. Wellness culture has had an enormous role in creating a lack of trust in our bodies. The messaging of the wellness industry has reinforced the idea that we are broken and we need to buy their cure to fix us. When we buy into this as truth, we experience something called learned helplessness, a psychological state in which we accept a perceived lack of control instead of fighting against it.

My client David grew up in a house where sweets were locked up, and seconds at meals were forbidden. Every food in the fridge was monitored and accounted for, and his parents would dish out each meal and snack for him up until David was a preteen. It's just the way it was in his house.

When David came to see me, he was struggling with overeating and the feeling that he had no control over his appetite or food intake. He constantly felt as though he had to limit his portions, and tightly schedule every meal and snack. This was obviously because of the way he had grown up, but as an adult, he was unable to trust himself to buy and eat appropriate amounts of food and to eat freely without a schedule. He seemed constantly at odds with what his body was asking him for because he just couldn't reconcile that with his need to control everything he ate.

People who grow up with parents who felt as though they had to control every morsel of food in the house, including how much their kids ate at meals, sometimes didn't have the chance to learn what we call self-regulation. This means that as children, they relied on others to tell them what and when to eat, and as adults, they struggle to learn self-regulation because they were taught—either directly or indirectly—that they couldn't be trusted around food. This was David's main issue—his parents never let him develop his self-regulatory skills in terms of food choices and appetite, and the feeling that he couldn't trust his body's cues or his food choices became a negative core belief that was impacting his life greatly as an adult.

If your negative core belief is that your body can't be trusted to tell you what it wants, to show you when it's hungry and full, and to signal when it's satisfied, it's very difficult to reject diet culture. If you don't trust your body, it seems like a very big leap to stop dieting and even believe that you can eat normally without tracking and worrying about everything you put into your mouth. Together, we can change that.

Question whether this core belief is true.

Do you believe that wellness, diet culture, and others know more about your body than you do? Do you believe that you have no self-control or willpower? That your body can't be trusted, or that if you give it some slack, it will betray you? Or, that giving over the control of your body to a diet or schedule is going to help make everything right? What backs this up? I'll wait.

Flip your negative core belief into a positive.

For example, "I know what's best for my body, and my body knows what's best for it. In the past, it was the diets that failed me; I didn't fail the diets." Can you think of some reasons this is true? Remember, after dismantling the negative core belief, you need to bolster your positive replacement. And we definitely don't want to see this troll rearing its head again.

Question #5: Do you moralize your eating habits and food in general?

This is a biggie for me, just take the title of my book. Do you categorize food as good and bad, right or wrong? Do you categorize your food choices and behaviors as good and bad? What does perfection mean to you in terms of what you eat and your body? Where did these notions originate? Looking at them now, note your perceptions.

Core belief #5: I am my diet.

It's trendy to categorize food as good and bad or use the word "clean" to describe your diet or food choices. This is language that's often used by wellness influencers and companies, but ironically, it reinforces the common negative core belief that you are your diet.

So many of my clients tell me that they've been bad with their eating.

Alex was a young woman who came to me for some diet tweaks. Everything was going well in our session, but I noticed that she constantly made references to food and eating as being good, eating clean, or cheating. I pick that stuff up immediately in a client's talk because it's a dead giveaway that they have their wires crossed. And by wires, I mean the food wire and the morality wire.

When clients like Alex moralize their food, they're commenting on how they view themselves. And although it's usually off-the-cuff, it's an underhanded way of saying that what they've done is shameful. It's a short jump from "These Doritos are bad" to "I'm bad because I ate these Doritos."

The problem is that using morally charged expressions to describe your diet can breed guilt and shame. The terms are often used interchangeably, and while they can both apply to how somebody reacts to food, these emotions are actually different. Guilt is feeling remorse for an action that you believe is wrong. For example, "I *feel* guilty because I ate that cake." Sure, you might feel physically crappy because you've eaten too much, but to feel guilty because you've broken the rules perpetuates the idea that food is right or wrong. Shame is how we feel about ourselves after doing something that we feel is wrong. For example, "I *am* bad because I ate that cake." When we feel shame, we're feeling judgment about who we are as a person.

You may even say these things to yourself in your head multiple times a day without realizing it. By doing that, you're living by your core belief: You're not a good person if you don't eat the way you think you're supposed to. This can have a negative impact on your food choices and your mood, not to mention your feelings about your overall self-worth.

Food and morality aren't strangers. We've long associated pure and natural foods with superiority. Diet and wellness cultures elicit a fervor that mimics religion among some people, who shun "demons" (often sugar or gluten) and worship purity, which ostensibly comes from "clean eating." Followers feel as though they're part of a bigger cause and governed by doctrines that often become their identities. And the "I am my diet" core belief often goes hand in hand with the "I need to be perfect or I'm a failure" core belief. They're like best friends.

With Alex, this couldn't have been more true. Her drive for perfection in her work (just made partner at her firm!) and her personal life (had the BEST boyfriend ever!) was also reflected in her eating habits. I could almost feel her disgust with herself as she described how she went to a barbecue with her boyfriend the weekend before our session and cheated on her diet by eating an entire bowl of Chicago-style popcorn. She felt dirty and like a failure that she had been unable to resist that bowl of ultradeliciousness, so much so that she looked like she wanted to jump out of her skin. Instead, she talked about eating extra-clean for the week, not eating any sugar at all, and going to Whole Foods and buying bottles of green juice that she'd bring for her lunches.

Her compulsion to jump back from eating "unclean" food as though she had just touched a hot stove was concerning to me. It looked as though Alex was going down the path toward orthorexia, an eating disorder that involves an unhealthy obsession with healthy eating. The food must be good and your habits must be perfect, or you're a failure. One of my favorite sayings is, "In nutrition, there is no such thing as perfection." And I truly believe that with all my heart.

Just for a moment, consider what it would feel like to let go of the goal of eating "perfectly." Whatever perfection means to you, ask yourself if it would make you happy? Would it be sustainable? Are you miserable trying to achieve it?

Question whether this core belief is true.

Do you believe that who you are as a person is determined by what you eat? That people who don't eat clean or eat healthy foods are somehow lesser? Think about what proof you have that this is true. What's really behind your thinking?

Flip your negative core belief into a positive.

Try telling yourself, "What I eat has nothing to do with who I am as a person. Morality-based terms for food are irrelevant and damaging to my relationship with food and with myself."

Again, list the evidence that supports this new, positive core belief to strengthen your resolve and kick that negative one to the curb. How do you feel? Better, I hope!

ROUTING THE REST

There are many other negative core beliefs out there. They can be like whack-a-moles! To discover all your core beliefs, you'll have to probe your feelings in each food-related situation—like a kid who keeps asking "But why?"—until you arrive at your answer. You might "why" yourself almost to oblivion, but that's okay. Keep asking until you come down to the truth.

Then you'll need to explore and evaluate (and reevaluate) that statement with a string of related questions. Let's use a common trigger event as an example.

watch out:

for "should."

"Should" is a red flag word. When we say the word "should," we are using judgment to motivate ourselves to be something different. For example, "I should be thinner. I should be able to handle this way of eating." When was the last time being judged resulted in positive, lasting change? Yeah, probably never. By should-ing ourselves, we are breaking our spirit.

Think about how often you tell yourself you should do or be something different. Then ask yourself why you're feeling that way. And who says? Is the voice you're hearing yours or somebody else's? List the reasons why they get a say in who you are and how you behave. Are they legitimate reasons?

Remember: You don't owe your life and well-being to anyone but yourself. If you don't fit somebody else's vision for you, they can piss right off. Nobody has any right to tell you how to be, how to look, and how to feel.

You go out for dinner with friends and end up overeating and feeling guilty, but your friends are all enjoying their food. The core belief here is: "I should feel guilty about eating the wrong things in the wrong amounts." Now start questioning that belief. That might go something like this:

Q: Why do you feel guilty about eating certain foods?
A: Because they're bad for me.

Q: Do you think that's really the case? Are certain foods going to ruin your health if you enjoy them occasionally?
A: Well, I know that they're not healthy to eat all of the time.

Q: But you don't eat them all of the time, and even if you did, what do you think would happen?
A: I'm afraid of gaining weight.

Q: Okay, so you're afraid. What is it about gaining weight that's making you afraid?
A: Because I'll get fat and feel like a failure.

Q: Is that a rational belief? Do you really think it's possible that you will gain weight from one meal or by eating certain foods some of the time? And does weight gain equal failure?
A: Well, probably not.

Q: How is this belief impacting your quality of life?
A: It's making me anxious and distracting me from important things, like time with friends and family.

Q: Do you truly believe that how you look determines what sort of person you are, or is that somebody else's idea?
A: I guess I don't really believe that my weight and appearance say who I am as a person. But my mom was always dieting in front of me and I think I just grew up thinking that eating unhealthy food and gaining weight makes me less of a person. At least, my mom was always making it seems as though that was the case.

Q: And what do you have to gain if you allow yourself to reject what's essentially your mother's old core belief and shed the guilt of enjoying these certain foods?
A: I think it would be a lot more fun and relaxing to be with my friends if I wasn't obsessing about everything I was ordering and eating.

Q: And do you think you deserve to have that experience?
A: I do.

Q: Okay, so are you ready to rethink your original belief: "I should feel guilty about eating the wrong things in the wrong amounts"?
A: Yes. How about, "Feeling guilty when I eat certain foods really diminishes the pleasure I get from eating and being with my friends. I deserve that pleasure, and there is absolutely no reason why I shouldn't have it. Even if I gained weight, it would never change who I am as a person."

There you go. Continue to reinforce this new positive core belief with proof that you gather over time. Repeat it to yourself. Write it down. Live it.

QUIETING THOSE VOICES

Tackling your negative core beliefs is an important step, but you may still have damaging thoughts from time to time. This is totally normal. The harmful self-talk goes hand in hand with negative core beliefs. Just remember that thoughts about yourself that make you feel unworthy, unhappy, shameful, or guilty are bullshit at best and harmful at worst.

Some of the common "thought invaders" my clients often report hearing in their heads are: "I'm so fat." "I can't lose weight." "I have no willpower against food." If these unwelcome statements enter your mind, ask yourself: If anyone—a friend, your child, your coworker—said this to you, would you agree? Would you say this to someone you care about? The answer is so often no. So what makes it okay for you to say it over and over again, day after day, year after year? Exactly. You don't deserve this kind of treatment.

It's time to examine our disdain for "fat" and put it to rest. Why are we so afraid of it? Is that logical? Like Beyoncé's scale-stepping video, is weaponizing the word "fat" really fair? Is it serving us, and others? This is a systemic issue in our culture that I'm not going to change here, but if you can start to really think about this word and shift your feelings about it, that's a win in my book.

What I want is for you to learn to slam the window down on these creepy little thoughts every time they try to crawl into your mind. Here are some other ways you can quiet those thoughts.

- ✕ Write a letter to the voice. If talking back to your voices doesn't do it for you, write them a letter. Tell them exactly what you think of them, and why you deserve to be successful and healthy. Tell them how they make you feel, and why they're not worth listening to. Describe how your life will be so much better without them, and how you're not going to let them in anymore. They're not welcome here.

- ✕ Journal your feelings. Keeping our stuff bottled up inside just lets it fester. Get it out and into a journal where you can keep track of your challenges and successes. Journaling can help you see things objectively. It can also help with working out your feelings, where they came from, why they're upsetting you, and the progress you make with them.

Working through negative core beliefs is a process that takes time. Keep at it, and don't give up! We've done a lot of work here, and you've done great things. Even the act of starting to address these issues, and face them once and for all, is a monumental step in the right direction. Please recognize that and know that this is a road that will lead you to a greater understanding of who you are and why you make the choices you make, think the things you think, and do the things you do. Good or bad, tough or easy, this is valuable information to have. And I commend you for taking this first step.

As we continue along our journey together, if you feel as though you need to revisit this chapter and address your negative core beliefs again, go ahead and do it. My expectation is that you'll need to refresh and reset your relationship with yourself and with food more than once. And remember: Talking about things can help immensely. Make sure you lean on any supports you have during this time.

In the meantime, let's move on to the next part of our journey: hunger.

know your hunger

I can't believe I'm even saying this, but hunger has become a battlefield as of late. Some people deny their hunger in the name of weight loss. Others think of hunger as a sign of weakness. Me? I see hunger throwing people into a tormenting spin: "What do I eat? What should I not eat? How much? How often?"

Eating is something we do every day. It should be second nature, but unfortunately for many people, it's not. The very act of choosing food has become a war zone within ourselves. And the truth is, true hunger is a cue that our body throws us when it needs food. And like other internal cues, it should be listened and attended to. In this chapter we're going to walk through normal eating, fullness, satisfaction, and the different types of hunger.

WHAT IS NORMAL EATING?

We all know how to eat, but eating and *normal eating* aren't the same thing and many of us have forgotten what the latter feels like. We often mistake normal eating with choosing the "right" foods. But as you know by now, there are no right and wrong food choices. It's entirely "normal" to occasionally overeat or to choose foods that are highly pleasurable to most of us, but not the most nutritious. In other words, it's normal for us to sometimes choose chocolate over salad, and that's okay.

Normal eating looks like this:

- ✂ Eating in a consistent and sustainable way.
- ✂ Understanding that sometimes we overeat.
- ✂ Feeling hunger when we start eating and feeling satisfied when we stop.
- ✂ Choosing foods that most often support our long-term physical and emotional health.
- ✂ Eating a wide variety of foods.
- ✂ Feeling peace, not guilt and shame, around food.
- ✂ Understanding that on some days, we'll need more food. On others, we'll need less.

Those are my guidelines for normal eating and they promote not only physical, but emotional wellness. Now, for contrast, let's talk about what normal eating is not:

- ✂ Restricting entire food groups for the sake of a diet (e.g., not eating fruit because the diet says it's bad).
- ✂ Putting your trust in anyone who tells you to eat a certain

way, but can't back their recommendations up with science.

- ✗ Ignoring your body's cues around eating or thinking it's wrong when you feel hunger.
- ✗ Constantly counting calories.
- ✗ Eating only avocados or celery juice or some other food selectively.
- ✗ Feeling forced to eat foods you dislike or that make you ill because your diet calls for them.
- ✗ Binge eating.
- ✗ Eating tiny amounts and walking around starving all the time.
- ✗ Having guilt and berating yourself about finding pleasure in food.
- ✗ Feeling shame about the food you eat or the amount you've eaten.
- ✗ Obsessing about what you eat before, during, and after you eat it.
- ✗ Constantly talking about food.
- ✗ Feeling like you can't trust your body around food.
- ✗ Ignoring your cravings and relying on willpower instead.

Whoa, that's a long list! Sadly, I see people doing these things on a daily basis.

I wouldn't be surprised if you found yourself identifying with a bunch of things on both lists. Or thinking that normal eating is actually harder than you thought it would be. It is harder, and that's because we've become so accustomed to eating with an agenda. An agenda has infiltrated our culture with constant messaging: Eat this, don't eat that. Eat to be thin. Don't gain weight. There's something wrong with your body. Starving yourself is a badge of honor.

Listen to this unqualified, full-of-shit "health guru." It's all garbage diet culture talk, and it's the end of the road for that crap.

Diet culture has changed our perception of what eating should look like. It has led us away from *picking up on our body's natural cues and instead made us reliant on external cues to tell us when and what to eat.* But only your body can tell you what it needs. No diet program, algorithm, or app can accurately predict how many calories you need in a day, how you process those calories, or when your body really needs to eat. We don't have the capacity to figure out our exact daily nutrient requirements, which can shift from day to day depending on our level of activity, hormones, environment, and myriad other factors. So when you're following that 1,200-calorie meal plan that your trainer or some diet app gave to you, you're not acting in tune with your body. You're using an external cue to give you information your body inherently already has. We need to listen to our bodies, not to our external cues, more often.

Here's the ugly truth: Diets oppose the natural forces at play in our bodies, and anyone who has been on a diet can attest to how bad—physically and emotionally—that can feel. Physically, you feel hungry and unsatisfied. Emotionally, you're cranky, frustrated, and fragile. Think about the last time you were on a diet.

- ✖ Did you eat when you were hungry (and I don't mean hungry as being starving from restricting food)?
- ✖ Did you choose foods that you wanted to eat, not foods that you were told to eat?
- ✖ Did you eat more because you had leftover calories you were instructed to consume?
- ✖ Did you ignore your hunger cues because you had expended your calorie allowance or it didn't fit into the diet's restrictions?

My bet is that you pretty much ate the food you were told to eat, at the times and in the quantities you were allowed to. You looked to the diet for cues about when and what to eat rather than tuning in to what your body was trying to say to you.

If you let it, diet culture will take away your power when it comes to food. It will convince you that your body can't be trusted, and that you're incapable of managing your eating on your own. It uses fear to reinforce those assertions, because there's big money to be made in convincing you to give over your power in order to be a loyal lifetime follower.

I want you to be able to step away from controlling diets and toward a more balanced way of eating. Normalizing your eating habits by listening to what your body needs can bring you emotional peace and physical satisfaction, and help repair your relationship with food by putting the responsibility for your choices squarely in your own hands.

If you've been dieting and restricting the amounts and types of food you eat for a while, you might not remember what hunger feels like. It's completely normal (although not necessarily a good thing) to lose your internal cues when you've been overriding them with random calorie and macro allowances, an eating schedule, prescriptive food lists, and everything else that diets are about. Basically, you've been following everyone else's rules but your own! So when it comes to nutrition and eating, we need to get you back in touch with your body so you're listening to nobody else but you.

Let's start by learning about hunger.

TRUE HUNGER

Babies eat when they're hungry and stop eating when they're full. This is *true hunger* and it's a physical feeling, not an emotional one.

Hunger and fullness are innate cues that we're born with. Just like you wouldn't ignore the urge to pee, you shouldn't be ignoring your true hunger. We need to nurture those cues and listen to them.

Eating when you're truly hungry can help stabilize your weight, mood, and hormones. And while emotional eating may be used to satisfy other needs, only the eating we do in response to true hunger can result in both physical and emotional satisfaction.

FALSE HUNGER

So what happens to that intuition? As we grow, outside influences sometimes override our natural instincts. For example, if my stomach grumbles but my diet tells me that I'm not allowed to eat yet, I'm going to wait to have lunch. This kind of conditioning can lead to false hunger, eating when we're not truly hungry.

Sometimes, our brains tell us to eat even if we're not hungry. For instance, if you put a piece of chocolate cake in front of me, I'm probably going to eat it because it looks good, even if I'm not hungry for it. This is called *visual hunger*. Visual hunger is wanting to eat not because you're hungry, but because you see food that looks good. It could be donuts in the break room after lunch at work or fries on your friend's plate after you've finished your own meal. Visual hunger can also be associated with situations that remind you of food, like watching a cooking show on TV, smelling popcorn at the movies, or seeing an ad for a delicious-looking burger.

Cravings are completely separate from hunger. They're classified as "hedonic responses to food," meaning that we crave something that is pleasurable and fun. This is why we generally end up craving chips or cupcakes versus salad and chicken breasts. We also tend to crave things that we're restricting or that we believe are off-limits to us. Which means, when we are on a restrictive diet, we tend to crave the foods we aren't allowed to eat. And we have plenty of research to confirm it.[1, 2, 3]

There's a school of thought that our bodies crave what we need, but research doesn't confirm this theory, except in the case of pica, in which pregnant women in need of minerals eat clay, chalk, and other inedible things. What's more likely is that our cravings result from emotional or hormonal triggers, which we'll cover more in Chapter 5. Some research has attempted to pin our cravings on our gut bacteria, but we still have very limited knowledge about this theory.[4]

A few things do diminish cravings. First, letting yourself have what you're craving eliminates that forbidden fruit syndrome of wanting what you can't have. You may initially overeat what you've been withholding, but eventually, it will become another food to you.

Some people aren't comfortable having certain foods hanging around their house, and I get it. There are some foods that I know I'm going to overeat, plain and simple. So, I limit the times that I have them in the house, which are few and far between. Do I let myself eat them without guilt and shame? For sure I do. If I want them, do I go and get them? Yup. But I find that having them in my face is sometimes just too much.

I don't look at this as a form of restriction but rather as a form of awareness. Science shows that some of us respond to external cues to eat more than others. Again, this is normal, but not ideal. I want you to enjoy these foods because you're truly hungry, not because of an outside influence. Recognizing visual triggers and removing them is one way to help accomplish that.

There's also *emotional hunger*, which is related to emotional eating. Many of us picture emotional eating as the quintessential pint of ice cream to nurse ourselves through a bad breakup, but in fact, emotional eating can be in response to all emotions—happiness, anger, sadness, anxiety, excitement. It's not necessarily associated with only bad emotions.

I've had plenty of clients who have struggled with visual or emotional hunger and didn't even know that they were being influenced by outside cues.

CASE STUDY: THE EMOTIONAL EATER

Paul had a pretty stressful life. He was the VP of a large company and under a lot of pressure to keep everything running smoothly. He traveled a lot for work and had a brutal commute, but the highlight of his day was coming home to his family.

"I love coming home to my kids and my wife," he told me. "But I literally eat all night long, starting from about half an hour after I walk through the door."

He couldn't understand it—he didn't overeat or even have the urge to during the workday.

"Can you walk me through a typical evening at home?" I asked.

"When I get home, my wife is starting to make dinner. She's managed two of the three kids all day, sent the other off to school, then picked him up after, given them all snacks, and gotten groceries, so I take the kids while she finishes cooking. We eat as a family, and we generally enjoy that. But after, not surprisingly, my wife is exhausted. I take over caring for the kids at that point, playing with them and then putting them to bed while she has some time to herself.

"I guess when I cross through the front door each evening, I feel like my day just goes on and on. I don't get a real break between work and being with the kids, which I love, but it can be exhausting, too. To keep myself going, I pick at whatever is lying out on the counters,

I go into the candy jar we have in our living room, and I finish the kids' dinner plates and bedtime snacks. I know I'm not hungry and yet I can't seem to stop putting food in my mouth all night long."

"Sounds to me like you're emotionally eating," I say. "You've got a lot of responsibilities once you get home, and you're looking to food to give you the energy to keep going. Is it working?"

Paul sighs. "Not really. If anything, I feel lethargic, bloated, and burned out by about 9 p.m., probably from eating too much sugar after dinner. It feels like I'm filling up on junk when I should be trying to enjoy my family."

Paul had an important realization, so I let it sink in. He really was going from one stressful situation at work into another at home. He wanted to give his wife some well-deserved rest time, but that meant he didn't have any for himself. And to compensate, he was eating out of stress.

Once Paul was aware of his own stress triggers and why he was overeating, he talked with his wife, and together they rearranged evening chores so that they both got a bit of individual time for peace and relaxation. With their new arrangement in place, he was able to name his feelings and filled the void not with empty consumption but with some "me time."

What can we learn from Paul? His pattern of mindless eating was unrelated to hunger; it was a result of emotional hunger. He was filling himself with food instead of what he really needed—a little bit of time to himself to de-stress and regroup. Once he became aware of this, it was easier to change his behavior and to start listening to true physical cues of hunger.

Paul's issue isn't uncommon. We all eat emotionally sometimes. If it happens often—several times a week or more—and you're using food as your primary coping mechanism, this can have a negative impact on your emotional and physical health. It's important to get to the reasons why you're using food to cope and then find other coping methods. Whether that's getting out and moving your body, talking to someone, writing, or creating art, there are other options. I personally find it tough to exercise when I'm anxious because my anxiety is so distracting. But walking does help me sort out my feelings because it gets me outside, which decreases my stress. Everybody's different, so you'll need to find what nonfood coping mechanism works best for you.

I'm here to help you do all of that. One of the first things we need to do is learn how to recognize the difference between true hunger and false hunger.

THE HUNGER AND FULLNESS SCALE

When you're learning (or relearning) what true hunger feels like, it can be helpful to use a scale to score your hunger levels. Over time, doing this can tell you important things about your true hunger, such as:

- ✗ How you feel when you're hungry. Some feel hunger in their stomachs, others simply get irritable and tired when they need to eat.
- ✗ When the best times are for you to eat your meals. Lunch may be earlier or later than noon depending on the day or what you've had for breakfast. For example, if you eat a high-protein breakfast, you might not feel hungry until 1 p.m. If you skip breakfast or eat something small, you might be hungry earlier. Your body will let you know.
- ✗ How you feel when you're perfectly satisfied versus how you've felt after meals when you were dieting.
- ✗ What true hunger, satisfaction, and fullness feel like.

Think of the hunger and fullness scale as numbers from 1 to 10.

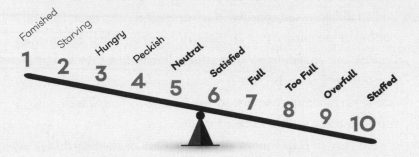

1 = **Famished.** This is the hungriest you can get. You're jittery, sweaty, probably faint, and your energy is flagging. You don't want to do much of anything except find food.

2 = **Starving.** You're having trouble concentrating and you feel weak. You're irritated or hangry. Your stomach is empty and growling. If you're a chronic dieter, you might be very familiar with how it feels to be a 2 on the hunger and fullness scale.

3 = **Hungry.** Your stomach is starting to growl. You might feel tired and less energetic. You should think about eating.

4 = **Peckish.** You're getting hungry.

5 = **Neutral.** The sensations of hunger are abating and you're in the middle of hungry and full. If you're a chronic dieter, you'll be used to stopping eating here.

6 = **Satisfied.** You're beginning to feel satisfaction in the form of warmth and fullness. You could eat more, but you're also fine as is. If you stopped now, you might be hungry in a couple of hours.

7 = **Full.** You're comfortably full and you feel expansion in your belly. You could probably eat more, but you don't need to. Your energy is up, and you're mentally sharp. You're satisfied and there are no signs of hunger to be found. This is when you should stop eating.

8 = Too Full. You're slightly uncomfortable; you could have eaten less. If you often withhold food from yourself or skip meals, when you do eat, you might find yourself coasting right by an 8 and into uncomfortable 9 or 10. This happens simply because you're so hungry, you're probably eating fast, and you may be in feast versus famine mode.

9 = Overfull. You're not feeling too good. Your stomach is bloated and achy, and your clothes feel a bit tight.

10 = Stuffed. This is the fullest you can be without actually throwing up. Your stomach feels painful and stretched, and you feel nauseous and sick. You probably don't want to do anything but lie down.

Ideally, you'd eat when you're between a 3 and 4 on the hunger scale, and stop when you're between 6 and 7. But some days you might be in a meeting and unable to get to lunch until late. Maybe you're traveling and you're stuck on a plane without anything to eat and there's no food in sight. You might overeat if you've let yourself get too hungry before your next meal or you're at a family celebration. The ideal isn't always possible—shit happens!—but the purpose of the hunger and fullness scale is to learn to recognize when you're truly hungry.

DEALING WITH VISUAL HUNGER

If you're not truly hungry but feel the need to eat because of a visual cue, acknowledge the feeling. If you really want what you're seeing, eat it and get over it. Obsessing over your choice isn't going to help you, and in fact, it could lead you down the path of overeating out of guilt. Repeat after me: Guilt and shame don't play nice with food and eating!

The best way to remedy visual hunger is to anticipate it and eat a nourishing meal beforehand. Ever hear the saying "Never go to the supermarket hungry"? This is the same idea. For example, if you know that you're going to the movies at dinnertime, have dinner first, and if you still want popcorn, order it. Don't sit through the movie salivating and distracted because you've told yourself that popcorn is off-limits.

Anticipate your visual hunger beforehand and manage it by eating a balanced meal and not making anything off-limits.

CASE STUDY: THE SNACKER

I had a client whose desk was in front of the office snack table, which led her to have snacks on the brain all day long. She told herself that she wasn't allowed any sweets at all, but she always ended up eating them anyway. This was disrupting her health because she was eating a lot of sweets and had gained a significant amount of weight just from that behavior.

The solution? Multipronged.

She started eating protein-rich meals and snacks to help curb her hunger, and got permission to move her desk away from the snack table. She also gave herself the go-ahead to eat snacks, so they weren't off-limits. This immediately made them less attractive to her.

But because life isn't always predictable, sometimes anticipating visual hunger will be impossible. That's totally fine! Do your best. You'll eat out of visual hunger sometimes, and that's totally okay. But if you're finding that visual cues are frequently influencing your choices over your true hunger, you may want to ask yourself the emotional hunger questions below. And if you need more help around the psychological triggers you have related to eating, a professional therapist can help.

DEALING WITH EMOTIONAL HUNGER

You might find it helpful to make a hunger journal. Grab a note-book and use it to track your hunger to get a better handle on when you're eating and why. When you feel like you want to eat, score your hunger on the hunger and fullness scale, and jot it down in the journal. Include the time of day and any emotions you may be feeling at the time. If you score between 7 and 10 on the hunger and fullness scale but you still feel like eating, explore what you're really feeling at the time in your journal. Are you stressed? Sad? Happy? Anxious? Nostalgic? Afraid?

When we eat because of emotional hunger, we're merely putting a Band-Aid on our feelings. This can feel good at the time if you're distracting yourself from something unhappy, but when the high of eating wears off, you're in the same place as before. As we discussed back in Chapter 2, getting to the bottom of our feelings can be tough and shitty, but it helps us move forward.

When you identify that you are emotionally hungry, ask your-self these questions:

- ✕ What is this emotion? Am I hiding it behind food?
- ✕ Why am I feeling this way? Say or journal it to yourself. So if you say, "I'm really sad," take it further. Why are you sad? Call that emotion out! "I'm sad because X." When you shine a light on what's truly bothering you instead of stuffing it down with food, you can get rid of it.
- ✕ What can I do about this emotion? Do you need to speak to someone? Could you take a walk, go for a swim, or journal about it some more?
- ✕ If I eat in response to this emotion, how will that make me feel? In some instances—especially happy ones—you'll eat

and feel good about it and that's great. But in instances when you're trying to cover up other, less happy emotions, you may not feel relief from eating. Acknowledge this.

THE DIFFERENCE BETWEEN SATISFIED AND FULL

As you listen to your body more, you'll recognize your real hunger cues. Once you have a sense of what true hunger feels like, you can start to differentiate between feeling full and feeling satisfied after a meal.

While there are different degrees of fullness, as you saw with the hunger and fullness scale, in general, *fullness is the sensation of having eaten enough or more than enough.* If you're a chronic dieter, feeling full might make you feel guilty and feeling hungry might make you feel like you're accomplishing something. This is diet culture knocking, so don't answer the door. Feeling full is a good thing; there's nothing wrong with it.

Sometimes, though, you can be full but not satisfied after a meal. Satisfaction is not only physical, it's also psychological. *Satisfaction comes from eating foods we enjoy.* A lot of us feel as though we aren't supposed to enjoy food, but this is just more diet culture bullshittery. Of course we're supposed to enjoy food! While some of us will find more pleasure in eating than others—where are my foodies at?—overall, eating should never be a negative experience. If a diet is too restrictive, our meals won't feel satisfying and we may find ourselves feeling deprived, thinking about food all the time, and foraging around for more.

We've all been there. In the 1990s, I was obsessed with eating everything fat-free or low-fat. When low-fat Oreos came out, I ran to the store to get them. I ate a ton of them, but still wanted more. They were so unsatisfying, I might as well have been eating sugared cardboard (actually, that's what they tasted like, too). I should have just eaten the whole-fat ones, which would have satisfied me more. Eating to feel satisfied means choosing and enjoying foods we like without guilt.

Above all else, meals should be nourishing and satisfying. This is normal eating and it takes care of our physical and emotional health.

WILLPOWER AND PERFECTION ARE MYTHS

The word "willpower" often comes up in diet culture, and the very word and what it represents in dieting makes me want to scream. The prevailing belief is that if you can't follow a diet, it's not the diet's fault: It's yours. You're weak, you're flawed. On the flip side, someone who is able to abstain from eating the wrong foods is strong. They are worthy of praise and recognition. They have willpower.

The perception that willpower has anything to do with eating and weight loss is not only preposterous, it's also physiologically unsound. In order to embrace a new view of normal eating, we have to let go of the idea that willpower has anything to do with healthy eating habits.

You see, when we're dieting, the drive to eat is mostly mediated by hormones, which are triggered by restriction and undereating. We are powerless when faced with our biological mechanisms. In other words, when you restrict your food intake, your body goes into red-alert mode. It doesn't like to be starved, and will do basically everything it can to get you to eat. There is no amount of willpower that can stand up to that natural force, so when we obey that call for food, nutrients, and energy, then feel guilt afterward because we lacked willpower, the diet industry wins. The truth? We never stood a chance.

Here's how it works.

Ghrelin, which is made in our stomach, is sometimes called the hunger hormone because it drives our appetite. When your body needs fuel, your ghrelin levels rise, and you can't focus on anything else but what you want to eat. You know the feeling: You've been on a diet for a few days, and everything looks delicious? That's the ghrelin talking, telling you to eat something already! Lack of sleep can also spike ghrelin levels, which accounts in part for that carb craving many of us have after we pull an all-nighter. Let's just say that when my daughter was born, I ate a *lot* of Starbucks apple fritters. My ghrelin was probably off the charts from lack of sleep and from exertion. Once you eat and your body no longer thinks it's in starvation mode, your ghrelin levels drop.

Leptin is a hormone produced by fat cells, and it keeps your brain up-to-date on your body fat reserves by telling your central nervous system if you need to eat more or less. There are theories that say that leptin helps burn fat, but this has never been proven in humans. In fact, when anyone starts talking about "fat-burning hormones," I know they're full of shit. If any hormones burned fat the way these people say they do, don't you think we'd be injecting them all over the place?

If you have enough body fat, your leptin levels stay the same or rise, causing you to eat less. If you go on a diet and lose body fat, leptin levels fall, increasing your appetite. What's that about willpower again? You're pretty much powerless against leptin.

But wait! If someone has a lot of body fat, wouldn't their leptin levels be higher? And if so, wouldn't those high leptin levels result in a lower appetite? Unfortunately, no. When we reach a certain level of body fat, signals from both leptin and ghrelin get messed up. Our leptin levels are high, but the brain becomes resistant to leptin and doesn't hear it anymore when it tells our body to eat less.

Instead, the brain thinks we're not getting enough food because it's not getting the signals from our circulating leptin, and our appetite is stimulated, causing us to eat more than we need to. As we gain more fat, more leptin is produced, but again, the signal is blocked. It's a vicious cycle. Meanwhile, in the same situation, it doesn't take as much ghrelin to spark hunger, so we get an appetite more easily that way, too.

The overall message? *Cheating your body out of adequate calories will backfire each and every time, no matter how dedicated you are to a diet.*

Here's another example. I see a lot of clients with an all-or-nothing mentality, and when they restrict their food, it always causes more damage because their bodies come up with ways to get them to eat—through visual hunger, cravings, or emotional hunger. Then this happens: "I ate one piece of cake, so now that I've blown it, I might as well eat the whole cake, and whatever else I'm normally not allowed to eat." They binge and their eating gets out of control—that's not normal eating. This all-or-nothing thinking is the supreme saboteur of happiness and a nourishing diet, and it stems from the pressure of diet culture to be perfect.

Even if you think you can achieve what you believe to be the perfect diet, which would lead you to the perfect weight, consider the consequences. Will that process be miserable? Will it be sustainable? And consider the reason why you even believe that perfection is possible. Is diet culture telling you what you should be thinking, eating, and weighing?

Whatever your version of a perfect diet is, you'll be better releasing it into the universe, and instead adopting my philosophy that in nutrition, there is no such thing as perfection. Trying to achieve it can take years of happiness away from you for no return whatsoever. Accepting that perfection is not possible can defuse a tremendous amount of the pressure we put onto ourselves to eat or look a certain way—let's face it, it's usually both. Make peace with it: You'll never be perfect, nor should you want to be.

There are always outliers who can restrict food and lose weight for the long term, but in general, it's a miserable existence. These people give up a lot socially, emotionally, and physically to achieve this, and very few of us would find those sacrifices worth the outcome. You want to live your best life because life is short. That doesn't necessarily mean overeating every day, but it does mean feeling full *and* satisfied and enjoying food, friends, family, and all of the other things we lose when we diet.

Remember, normal eating is not about willpower or perfection, it's about listening to your body. Our bodies are a lot smarter than we often give them credit for. Willpower is no match for biology. And anyone who tells you different is wrong.

TRUST YOURSELF, TRUST YOUR BODY

As we saw in Chapter 2, many chronic dieters don't trust themselves around food. Food is the enemy that's out to tempt them, and they need to restrict how much and which foods they eat so they don't lose control. But by now we know that the tighter we hold on to that control, the less control we actually have and the worse we feel.

It's time to learn to trust yourself around food. This is an important step to healing your body. Here are some exercises you can do to build trust in yourself:

- ✖ If you have a trigger food that you obsess about all of the time, give yourself permission to eat it. Actually go ahead and eat that food and enjoy it. Do this every day if you need to.
- ✖ If you're worried about how much weight you think you're

going to gain, don't. Think of all the times you've restricted this food and then binged on it.

- When you eat this food, be aware of how it tastes and how it makes you feel physically. This is a mindfulness exercise. Don't sit in front of the TV or otherwise distract yourself while you're eating. Pay attention to the experience of pleasure. Pay attention to any physical signals your body sends regarding satisfaction or when you've had enough.

Emotionally, this exercise might be tough for some people. But what I'm trying to do is give you permission to enjoy a food that you've told yourself you have no right to enjoy. That alone may be enough for you to reawaken your body's physical sensations about when you're satisfied and normalize your eating. It may take a few tries, but over time, you'll likely find that your cravings toward a single food diminish once you allow yourself to have it. Eventually you might not even crave this food anymore.

I hope this chapter has helped you learn what it truly means and feels like to be hungry, full, and satisfied, and rethink your relationship with food, eating, and your body. This is all part of learning how to eat normally. It isn't easy, but it's the first step to finding peace. Go over the questions and exercises in this chapter as often as you need to. Do the hunger journal. Remember to ask yourself where your feelings are coming from. Talk about food and eating in positive terms only. Imagine a life where you don't feel guilty about food or strive for perfection.

You'll get there, and once you do, you'll be able to turn your back on diets forever.

map your goals

No matter what your goals are, your chances of success will be far higher if you're prepared for the work it takes to achieve them. That includes having a true picture of where you are now, where you want to end up, and the road between the two points. You've probably read a lot of diet books that list what you can and can't eat, give you a meal plan, and tell you to get started. Good luck. But this isn't one of those lame books. Hell no. This book is for keeps, and what you learn are skills that will last you a lifetime, not just a couple of months. Before we get into the practical work—the science of food and how to eat for health and satisfaction—we need to lay some groundwork.

When I was learning to drive, I had an instructor who was a bit weird, but he did end up teaching me two very important things:

✕ How to drive reasonably well (though my husband might dis-
agree).

✕ Not to accelerate into a place that you can't see, like around a
corner.

A lot of people want to make changes to their eating and lifestyle habits, but they just grab a couple of goals out of thin air and
hit the accelerator without mapping out a route. In other words,
they haven't taken into consideration their current lifestyle, their
wants and needs, their likes and dislikes, and their priorities to determine how their goals fit into their daily life. In a short time,
they're whipping around the bend, full speed ahead, toward a crash
that puts them right back where they were before they stepped into
the car. Except maybe more physically and emotionally banged up.
That, too.

How we eat and the food choices we make ripple out to all the
corners of our life: our relationships, our kids, our work, and our fi-
nances. That means that *the way we eat needs to fit with our lifestyle*,
but many people do the opposite and build their life around their
diet instead. They hear about a new diet that sounds amazing and
jump right into it without considering if it's consistent with their
values or how it will affect them and the people around them. If
the way you eat doesn't fit your lifestyle, it's going to be a miserable
time. And just as important, you'll never be able to sustain it.

This impulsive decision making can result in diet flip-flopping
forever. Go on a diet for a little while, realize that it's not a good
fit, go off that diet. Jump onto another diet, realize it's not a good fit,
go off that diet. Repeat X years of your life. Sound familiar?

If you're going to make lasting, meaningful change, you need to
do an assessment first. It's like a business plan: You list your current
situation, the cost benefit of your goal, how you're going to achieve

it, and how you're going to maintain it. Basically, I want you to set clear, achievable goals for yourself and visualize how you're going to meet them.

MAKE THE DESTINATION SPECIFIC

Let's start at the end. What are your goals? What do you want to achieve and why? Be specific.

You may have picked up this book because you want to lose weight. Or, you might be curious about nutrition. Or, you might want to eat a more nourishing diet. Whatever your reasons, we need to take a closer look at them. It's easy to say, "I'm reading this book because I want to lose forty pounds," but what exactly do you want to achieve by doing that?

I want you not to set an actual weight-number goal (this isn't a diet book, remember), but instead to *focus on what reaching your goals will bring you emotionally and physically*. For example, you'll be physically stronger and able to be more active with your kids. You'll have a better relationship with food, which will decrease your anxiety around eating. You'll be less confused about what to eat, and more organized and prepared for meals. You'll optimize your nutrition so you have more energy. You'll lose the urge to diet and be able to enjoy food without guilt or shame. You'll achieve a comfortable weight so you can enjoy life while still eating a variety of nourishing foods.

Instead of "I want to lose weight," your goal might now be, "I want to lose weight to help me feel more comfortable and be more mobile."

Doing this sort of work will help you break down your goal so you can visualize what your life will be like once you've achieved it. Setting a nebulous goal like "I want to lose weight" is too abstract, but being specific and descriptive forces you to really consider what you want and what it looks like.

One thing I want to caution against is setting specific number goals like "I want to lose ten pounds" or, "I am giving myself three months to lose weight." This isn't because I don't think any of that will happen. It very well might, but number goals are a diet culture trap.

A lot of fad diets tell people that they can lose X number of pounds in X time, but these number goals assume that we know exactly how our bodies are going to react to the changes we make, and in reality, we don't. You might lose seven pounds and feel good there. Or, losing weight might take longer than you expect. I don't have a crystal ball, and neither do you. Choosing specific number goals sets expectations that we don't know if you will be able to meet.

Remember, you're going for your comfortable weight, which means you can sustain it without a lot of hassle. It's a weight you maintain by making nourishing food choices most of the time but occasionally going out with your friends for steak frites or an ice cream sundae. It's not feeling like you have to punish yourself for what you've eaten.

MAKE THE DESTINATION YOURS

Are you setting this goal for you or for someone else?

Sometimes, we set goals for other people. For example, we want to fit into our high school jeans before the reunion because we want people to think we look good. Or, your mom told you that you're getting too heavy. Or, the all-too-common, "Diet culture said I'm fat so I guess I should lose weight, even though I feel good about myself." It's great to want to eat a more nourishing diet and most of us can make some tweaks, but embarking on a weight-loss journey because someone else wants you to is not okay. Not only does this cause major resentment toward that person (if their comments haven't done that already) and yourself, it makes any changes more difficult to sustain because they're not something you're really invested in for yourself.

Whatever your goal is, you need to do it for you. No matter what your size is, if you like the way you look, then everyone else can piss off. People who look at you funny or make ugly comments about your weight are projecting their shit onto you. Don't let them get away with it by submitting to their shaming.

MAKE THE DESTINATION REALISTIC

What expectations do you have around your goal? Are they realistic?

If you're expecting the ever-elusive "life transformation" that so many fad diets promise, I hate to break it to you, but that's not going to happen. Sure, if you change your eating behaviors and your relationship with food, your life will probably be better in a lot of ways. But you're still going to be the same person, with the same dust bunnies behind your bathroom door and the same boss you'd like to strangle. That shit's not going to change because of what you eat and how you feel about food. Remember, we talked about this in our negative core belief examples in Chapter 2.

It's important to *be flexible with your expectations*. Maybe you want everything to happen quickly. We're so conditioned to expect everything immediately—even I get itchy when a web page takes more than three seconds to load—but we need to learn to slow down. So, if you're looking to lose weight or make changes to your eating habits, don't give your body a deadline. That just sets you up for failure if you don't make the deadline. Remember, it's the emotional and physical gains that are important, not losing a certain amount of weight by a certain day or changing your habits overnight. Do it right, and let it take as long as it takes.

Changing your relationship with food is a process that takes time. A lot of us have grand expectations that when we change something, that change will be immediate and solid as a rock. But life isn't like that, and depending on the complexity of your relationship with food and your body, change can be tenuous at first. It needs to be nurtured and reinforced, supported, and repeated.

Some days, you'll feel good. You'll be cruising along with all of the new things we're learning here and you'll feel as though you're on the right track. But it's not always going to be that way. Some days, or weeks, will be like climbing a mountain. Life will hit you like a ton of bricks or you'll be triggered by something emotional, and you'll sink back into your old habits. But each time that happens, you won't sink as deep as the last until eventually, you'll bounce right up and dust yourself off.

Whatever your goals are, you need to be patient and flexible. Because they might happen just as you want them to, but they might not. If they do, I'm assuming you'd be stoked. If they don't, you should be willing to take a second look at your original goals and rework them to something that's still positive but more realistic. This doesn't constitute a failure. It doesn't mean you're weak or not disciplined; it just means that the goals you set didn't work for you.

Sometimes when we set goals, we over- or undershoot, so we need to be able to readjust and refocus. No biggie. Could you imagine a goal that's on a smaller scale than the one you've set? Write that goal down and keep yourself open to accommodating any twists and turns this road might take.

GET A GPS (AND A BACKUP MAP)

In other words, do you have support to help you along the way?

This is a big one. Embarking on a road trip without a GPS or even a map can be tough and it's the same with your journey toward your goal, whether that's eating more healthily or losing weight. Of course, you can do it on your own, but having people rallying around you, ready to offer a helping hand—like a map reader—makes the process smoother. *Don't be afraid to enlist support.*

For example, you might need someone to watch your kids so you can take that exercise class. Or, you might want to do a nourishing lunch exchange with some of your colleagues instead of going out to a restaurant. Having your family on board is especially good, since when you make changes to your eating habits, it's easier—and more sustainable—to make them to everyone's. I've counseled people whose significant other wasn't on board with their changes, and it was really hard on them. These people ended up finding support elsewhere.

Sometimes, that support comes in the form of a professional other than me. If you have a psychologist, psychiatrist, or counselor, they should know about the changes you're making. If there's somebody who has been helping you with your negative core beliefs, they'll be well versed in your story and can help you with emotional barriers or anything that might bubble up when you're on this journey. If you find that you're continually getting stuck with your eating and you believe that it's because of something emotional, I can't stress enough the importance of seeing a therapist. I can help you with food, but this book isn't a replacement for therapy.

So, who will your supports be? It's time to rally the troops and find your map readers!

LOOK UNDER THE HOOD

How would you describe your current diet?

You can't know where you're going and how you're going to get there unless you look at what exactly is happening right now in your life. Many clients tell me that they're comfortable with their current diet, but they think they need some tweaks. Others say they eat too much candy or fast food. Whatever you think of your current diet, I want you to make a list of the things you'd like to change. Maybe you want to eat more vegetables or start cooking more for yourself. Be gentle with yourself. You might be used to slashing stuff out of your diet, but that's not what this is about.

Aside from your goals, enjoying life is the object of the game. Do you really want to live in a world where you can't eat the foods you love ever again? I'll answer that for you. No, you don't. This isn't a diet book, and I don't operate from a place of absolutes. Remember: A nourishing diet involves all types of foods and is nourishing both physically and emotionally. I'm not going to tell you to cut out all the stuff you love. That's what diet culture does, and it tells us that the joy and meaning in our lives come down to one thing: thinness. So wrong.

You're reading this book for a reason, which means you probably want to change your diet in some fashion to achieve those goals we just set, so while I'm not going to remove anything from your diet, I will be asking you to make some changes as we move through the book together. Those might be to eat more of one food and less of another. You'll probably be eating the same volume of food, but maybe not all of the same types. At least, not as often.

Now that you've outlined your current diet and the things you want to change, the next step in your road map is to *write down the things that are negotiable and the things that are nonnegotiable.* Some people refuse to adjust the sugar or cream in their coffee. Others don't want to give up that glass of wine they enjoy a couple times a week. That's okay! We all have things we don't want to change. As long as you're open to making other changes to your eating habits and you're realistic—saying you want to drink a bottle of wine every night is not realistic—we can work around the nonnegotiables.

Your negotiables and nonnegotiables might change over time, but having a list of them will help you focus in on which changes you want to make.

KEEP A SPARE TIRE

What are the potential barriers and setbacks?

Okay, so you've made changes that are consistent with your values and are doable, flexible, and substantial enough that you can maintain them no matter what. Great work. But shit happens. You go through a breakup. You go on a work trip that includes rich, indulgent networking dinners every night. *Even with the best-laid plans and the most thought-out goals, there will be setbacks.*

In the past, you may have let flat tires, breakdowns, and rough terrain throw you off course, but I don't want that to happen here. While some mishaps will be unavoidable—that's life—others can be avoided or at least blunted if you anticipate and prepare for them. This is an essential part of making long-term change. I want to set you up for success so you can manage whatever comes your way.

As we walk through the different kinds of barriers described below, think about which ones might be potential setbacks on your journey toward your goal and how you might prepare for them. Some of what we consider to be setbacks might be better called learning experiences. Read on.

GEOGRAPHICAL BARRIERS

A lot of barriers are geographical. For example, you're away from home in a place where you don't have a lot of choice about what you eat, whether that's on vacation or a business trip or at someone else's house for dinner. These situations can be a very real source of anxiety for people who are trying to heal a relationship with food and change their eating habits.

How do you manage this potential barrier? First, realize that you can't control everything. That's the way life goes. But nothing bad is going to happen if you eat a little differently than you normally would. So go ahead and make peace with the fact that sometimes you're going to overeat. You shouldn't be feeling stuffed every day, but sometimes eating to an 8 or 9 or even 10 on the fullness scale is going to happen. That's human nature and everyone does it. Not a big deal; just move on and go back to your normal eating habits after.

Remember, experiences are what make our lives great and some of these involve food. If you're on vacation in Italy, it would be scandalous to spend your entire trip trying to avoid the local food. Pasta? Of course! Gelato? Definitely. Instead of dancing around trying to find something healthier, enjoy the satisfaction of eating delicious food. Think about the nourishment and pleasure you'll derive from the foods you're trying, the places you're going, the company you're with. When you're over at someone else's house for dinner, go with it. Build memories, not useless, counterproductive food guilt that does nobody any good, ever. Stressing out over a meal or five is not worth it, on vacation or otherwise.

Here are some tips for eating well *and* enjoying your food when you're away from home:

Choose vegetables first and protein second.

When you're at a structured meal—one that you intend on having and sit down to enjoy versus something on the fly—go for vegetables and protein if you can. Of course, if you're in Texas and your meal is a big plate of barbecue, that's okay! The next time you get to sit down to a meal where you can order a salad or vegetables, try to do so. If you're at a business dinner and you want the steak, but feel like the shrimp cocktail would be healthier, have a small steak and load the rest of the plate with vegetables. This combination will fill you up and help satisfy you. If you want to add a baked potato, go ahead.

Be aware of your hunger.

If you're satisfied after your steak or your pasta, then maybe you don't order dessert. If you encounter a gelato place that looks amazing and you're full, maybe you go back another time or eat some—or all—of a small cup, and get over it.

Stay somewhere with a working minibar fridge or a kitchen.

This is one way to keep a bit of normalcy in your schedule because it gives you the ability to make some of your own meals. When I travel with my family for more than a week or so, we try to get a suite with a kitchen because the thought of being stuck in a hotel room with no snacks is just too much for us to bear. Is that wrong? I also love checking out supermarkets in different cities. The first thing I do is I hit the closest supermarket or drugstore that has a food section and I load my basket with a small cut-vegetable tray or a bag of baby carrots, a couple pieces of fruit, some nuts, oatmeal cups that I can make with boiling water, tons of yogurt, and whatever else I can find. If we have a kitchen, I buy breakfast and snack foods like the ones above, plus a loaf of bread, butter, salad greens, tuna, oatmeal, anything else the kids want, like chips, and beer for my husband. This gives us some options for meals so we aren't forced to eat in restaurants for three meals a day.

Stay active.

When you're on vacation, walk around as much as you can and try active site-specific fun like snorkeling, hiking, skiing, or anything else you enjoy. If you're away on business, choose a hotel with a lap pool or gym, or hit a spin class in that city, if your schedule allows. That being said, don't stress yourself out trying to be active, if what you need is to plant your ass on a lounge chair and chill the heck out. Coming back from a vacation more stressed out than you were when you went is *not* the goal.

Pack snacks.

Whether you're on vacation or just have a long commute, it's easy to find yourself stuck in transit—plane, car, bus—totally hangry. Try to have a snack before you leave or bring one with you to stave off hunger so that when you arrive at your destination, you're not so ravenous that you hoover the entire kitchen or overeat at your next meal.

ENVIRONMENTAL BARRIERS

There are also regular environmental barriers like a workplace that prioritizes food and/or booze. Sometimes it can feel like there's food everywhere, especially when a box of chocolates is literally staring at you from every flat surface in the office. Remember, repeatedly denying yourself something that you crave can only lead to stronger cravings. But if you're confronted by food at every turn, it can be a barrier to make positive changes to your diet. The trick? Choose your battles. Or should I say, your cookies.

For example, Christmas might mean there's food all over the place at your job. Do you eat it all every single day that it's there? Nope. Do you eat some of the stuff that you love and can't always get? Damn straight you do. And you don't feel one bit of guilt about it. Screw that! While you're eating, keep tabs on your hunger as well as your satisfaction. Will one cookie do the trick? Great. Do you need two to feel satisfied? That's fine, too.

In a workplace that has a food and booze culture, as so many do these days, you'll have to learn how to say no. Choose the events you reeeeally want to go to and bail on the ones you can live without. So, Thirsty Thursday might be a yes, and that impromptu meetup for drinks after work on Friday will be an "I'm washing my hair" sort of thing. I know it's tough when peer pressure is working against you, and it's important to be social, but trust me: You're probably not missing much when you decline yet another invite.

If you're going to make changes, you're going to need to prioritize these things. It's the same with food at work. Maybe you go out for lunch once or twice, and bring your lunch the rest of the time. Or, you go to the break room to celebrate someone's birthday, but you don't always have a piece of cake. Especially when it's the kind of cake that you don't even like.

don'ts:

bank calories.

When I was in nutrition school, we learned to tell people to bank their calories if they had a big food-related event coming up. So, if they knew they were going to have Thanksgiving dinner, we'd suggest that they'd eat less for days before to make up for the calories they were going to gobble down at the holiday table. Now that I think about telling people that crap, I want to cringe. We've come a long way since then.

I never suggest this anymore, because cutting calories in anticipation of an event does two things: It gives you a feeling of permissiveness—"I cut calories, now I can go wild!"—and makes you hungrier, both of which can lead to overeating. Eat normally leading up to the event, and try to stay in touch with your body's cues as much as possible during the event.

try to burn off calories that you've eaten.

A lot of people will hit the gym after a big meal, trying to repent for their sins. But your body doesn't really work that way. We can only use a certain number of calories every day from intentional exercise, and it's a lot fewer than you think. When you overexercise, all you end up doing is make yourself hungrier, and again, there's a permissiveness that happens because you've "burned off the calories." It can lead you to develop a negative association toward food and toward exercise. The purpose of exercise is to strengthen your body and to release stress, not punish you.

EMOTIONAL BARRIERS

Some barriers are emotional. Sometimes, life throws uncomfortable situations at us that make us want to eat. You know what I'm talking about. Your boss gives you a ton of work to do . . . due tomorrow. Your girlfriend breaks up with you. Someone insults your weight or appearance. You fight with your mother-in-law.

I could list a million other examples, but you get the point. While we all have different tolerance levels, some of these scenarios can drive us to eat emotionally. Like I said earlier, this is a normal part of being human.

The problem is that when we use food as a coping mechanism, we weaponize it. Weaponizing food means using it against yourself, as in, "My boyfriend broke up with me, so I'm going to eat these two pints of ice cream to make myself feel better." You can also weaponize food to use against others, such as, "My aunt called me fat in front of everyone at the dinner table, so I'm going to eat twice as much now to show her that I don't give a shit about her opinions." Either option does you absolutely no good, and in the long run, you're more likely to feel worse than better, especially if you take it too far by overeating for an extended period of time, and you do not deserve to be punished for what somebody else does to you.

Instead of using food as a weapon, try to find other outlets for your emotions. Journaling. Activity. Movies. Something artistic. Speaking to a friend or therapist. Treating yourself with the love and respect you deserve.

HABITUAL BARRIERS

And lastly, barriers can be habitual. For example, going out to restaurants, ordering takeout, and eating prepared food instead of making your own meals. You can anticipate and manage all the barriers above, but you're just not used to doing that. Your habits are more of the Uber Eats sort of thing. But if you don't make time to prepare your own food consistently, you won't be able to properly nourish your body physically and emotionally, which is key to reaching whatever your goal is.

I get it. You don't feel like going all Martha Stewart. All that grocery shopping, prepping, freezing, ahhhh! It's easier just to order in from a restaurant. And yes, sometimes it is. But the truth is, relying on restaurant or prepared foods can be a real barrier to establishing better food habits. This is because you have zero control over what restaurants put into your food, so it's usually less nourishing than what you'd otherwise make for yourself. Portions from restaurants also tend to be larger, which may lead to you eating more out of visual hunger and the feeling of not wanting to waste what you've paid for.

If you have a family, preparing your own meals sets a great example for your kids and teaches them essential life skills like shopping and cooking. And let's face it: Prepared food is expensive. Think about what you could do with the money you save by cooking your own meals. Hello, Hawaii!

I hate to use absolutes with you, but I have to here. If you're going to successfully change your diet, you've got to make this one a priority. Don't worry—the key is to start small. Remember, big changes won't stick with your lifestyle, so we need to take baby steps. Here are some tips and tricks to help you:

- ✕ If you buy your lunch every day, try packing your lunch once or twice a week.
- ✕ If you normally grocery shop once every two weeks, set aside time each weekend to shop for the week. Do this every week.

- ✕ Never shop hungry.
- ✕ Make a list and consider your schedule for the upcoming week before you shop.
- ✕ After you do your shopping, batch-cook—we'll get into this in Chapter 9 on high-value eating.

The goal here is that you have readily available food that is delicious and nourishing so that when hunger strikes, you reach for these satisfying meals instead of the takeout menu.

Other barriers will pop up in the course of your life, but overcoming these hurdles here can be used to help you overcome those situations too. The key is to being prepared. So, are there any other potential barriers you foresee on your journey? How will you manage them when they arise? Write this all down.

So far, you've challenged your negative core beliefs and found your hunger cues (or at least, you know how to). You've learned about normal eating and the difference between being full and being satisfied. You're starting to get in touch with a new way of thinking not only about what you eat but what triggers your eating response. And now you've mapped out the road ahead, including all those pesky pitfalls waiting around the corners, so that your lifestyle works with your desired changes. For all of this, and for sticking with this journey, I want to congratulate you! YESSSS! Great job!

You're making progress, and you've truly laid a lot of the groundwork for a healthier relationship with food and eating. Now that you're on the right path, it's time to learn the basics of food. First stop? Carbs. Let's go.

#carbsarelife

Oh, carbohydrate. Everyone thinks you're such a naughty monkey, but you're just so misunderstood. Why?

Carbs have been vilified as of late because unlike protein and even more than fat, they come in forms that are highly refined, sugary, and easy to overeat: chips, crackers, cake, cookies, and all of the other things that people come to me complaining that they can't seem to get enough of. And overeaten them we have: Anyone who lived through the low-fat era in the nineties remembers how we took fat out of basically everything we could and replaced it with sugary carbs. During this time, Americans gained a lot of weight—not because of the carbs per se, but because we gave ourselves license to overeat everything that was fat-free. Fat was bad, and carbs of any kind? Good.

Now the pendulum has swung in the complete opposite

direction. We've come to love fat and fear carbs. Carbs—even fruit—have been accused of causing the rise in diabetes, obesity, allergies, and everything else that's wrong with us. But like a lot of what diet zealots say, this is a gross oversimplification of the truth.

Carbs don't deserve that entire burden. The rise in obesity and chronic disease isn't because people have eaten too much fruit or too much white bread. It has happened because of multiple factors: diets that consist mostly of highly refined foods, plus sedentary behavior, desserts, increased stress, less sleep, more store-bought meals and less home cooking, lack of access to services such as dietitians and physicians, as well as a lack of nutrition and home-economics education in schools. There is also the burden of choice, which rests on our shoulders. While some have little choice in what they eat, many of us do, and we've known for years that carbohydrates such as whole grains, fruit, and simply prepared starchy vegetables are the best choices for health versus their ultraprocessed counterparts. Still, we've freely chosen refined and ultraprocessed carbs instead of more physically nourishing ones, far too often. So yes, that's on us as a population.

Just because some forms of carbs are less nourishing than others doesn't mean that it's smart or correct to say that all carbs are bad. That's what we tend to do, though, because we're a culture of extremes that likes to label things as good or bad.

Thankfully, there is a happy medium, and even though the minutiae of that is different for everyone, overall it looks like this: some carbs. Not too many. Not too few. Mostly from whole sources. And a few Oreos along the way for me.

This chapter is going to help you take a new look at carbs: what they are, how many you should be eating, and why you shouldn't be afraid of them.

WHAT ARE CARBS?

Let's do a quick refresher. Carbohydrates are molecules found in food and are composed of carbon, hydrogen, and oxygen. Common foods high in carbohydrates are potatoes, grains, fruit, and sweets of all types. When we eat carbohydrates, our body breaks those molecules down into *glucose* or sugar, which is then shuttled from the bloodstream to the cells by the insulin that is released by the pancreas in response to a meal. In the cells, glucose is converted into energy for use right away, and if you don't need that energy right then, it's converted into *glycogen*, which is stored in the liver and muscles for later use. Most healthy people are well equipped to manage the metabolism of carbohydrate into glucose and glycogen, whether it's from oats or lollipops.

There is nothing harmful or unnatural about this process. We're so used to being told that carbs are harmful in some way, and they've shouldered that blame unnecessarily. Some people believe that the rise in insulin after we eat carbohydrates is dangerous. In reality, it's a normal, necessary physiological response that in healthy people has no negative effects. We need insulin to rise so that glucose gets to where it needs to be: in the cells. After that happens, insulin levels recede.

Carbohydrates are the first-line fuel for the brain and muscles, which I know is disputed by some low-carb dieters—more on them later—and people who like to ignore the rules of basic physiology. They like to talk about how we just don't need carbs at all. While we *can* live without them—our brain and muscles can turn fat and protein into glucose by a process called gluconeogenesis—that's not a good enough reason to take them out of our diet. There are a lot of nutrients to be found in many carbohydrates and they add so much satisfaction to our meals.

GUIDELINES FOR CARB INTAKE

How many carbohydrates do you need? I'm not going to tell you how many grams or calories' worth of carbs you'll need in a day, for two reasons. First of all, I have no idea. Everyone is different, and I'm not going to just throw random numbers out there as though you all need the exact same thing. That's what diet books do. Second, I want you to get away from counting shit, and giving you grams of this or calories of that works against this philosophy. I refuse to tell you exactly what to eat because we all know that that never works for the long term. What works is self-management, meaning you need to find out what's right for you. So, let's figure that out.

To get you started, here are some *loose* guidelines for nutrition and variety that most healthy people benefit from:

Protein and vegetables first, carbs next.

My recommendation is always to prioritize protein, then vegetables, then carbs. This hierarchy ensures your meals and snacks will be more satisfying and filling than if you started by filling your plate with carbs and then adding everything else.

One to three servings of fruits a day.

Don't listen to people who tell you to only eat green apples or berries because they're low in sugar. Fruit is fruit, and the differences in sugar content between different types is not going to make a significant impact on anything in your life provided you don't overindulge regularly. The truth is, that most people don't eat enough fruit to begin with, so choose whichever ones you love and enjoy them. A whole piece or a handful of berries or cut-up fruit is a serving.

A moderate amount of grains and starchy vegetables at each meal.

A moderate amount looks like a handful. So, half of a large baked potato, one or two pieces of bread, or a large spoonful of pasta. Fill a quarter of your plate with carbs at each meal and see how you feel with that amount. If you feel as though that's too much, try a meal or two without carbs at all. If you feel like your energy is low and you need more, bump up your servings a bit by half-cup increments. It's trial and error, and every day can be different. If you've been very active or intend on being very active, you may find you feel better with more carbs on your plate.

Although beans, lentils, and other legumes are carb-rich, they're considered to be protein foods. If your meal is based on legumes, scale back the other carbs on your plate by half, and fill the rest of the plate with vegetables.

A balanced approach to snacks.

It's easy to grab a piece of fruit or a couple of crackers for a snack, but because these things are mostly carbs, they're not as satisfying as when they're accompanied by a fat and a protein. So when you have a piece of fruit for a snack, add a piece of cheese or some nuts with it to amp up the satiety level. If you want to dial down the carbs, choose a lower-carb snack such as a couple of hard-boiled eggs, some avocado, and tomato mixed with oil and vinegar, or raw vegetables with hummus.

If you're having two to three snacks a day, I recommend having at least one or two of them be low-carb. Save the carb-rich one if you need something before your workout to give you an energy boost.

Desserts once a day.

If you love desserts, that's great—I do, too. Eat what you love. As we discussed earlier in the book, allowing yourself foods that you crave is part of a long-term approach to sustainable, nourishing eating. I tell clients to limit desserts to once a day in a reasonable portion. A small slice of cake. A couple of cookies. A small bowl of ice cream. Some days, you might find you don't want dessert at all, in which case you can skip it.

CARB TOLERANCE

The guidelines above are loose because I believe that everyone has a different carb tolerance, meaning some people can eat more carbs than others without gaining weight.

Your carb tolerance is mostly the result of genetics: Some people process carbohydrate better than others. Here's why: Salivary amylase is an enzyme that breaks down starch as soon as it comes into contact with our saliva. Some people have more salivary amylase, meaning that they break down starches better and faster than people who have less of this enzyme. Of course, salivary amylase is not the only factor that determines a person's weight. Activity level, medical conditions, and the type and amount of carbohydrate eaten are all factors.

The overall guideline in terms of carb tolerance is to eat enough carbs for you, without pushing it over the line. Everyone is different, but if you're looking to lose weight, then you want a carb level that allows you to lose and then maintain weight and energy levels while being active, happy, and satisfied both physically and emotionally. Notice that I say "lose and then maintain weight." No, I'm not confused—but think of it this way: Most diets instruct followers to drop carb levels drastically. This can result in weight loss, but it's often unsustainable, and when the person eventually starts to eat more carbs, they're unable to regulate the amount and so they regain that weight. If you figure out a sustainable, flexible carb level at the start of your journey, then along with other tweaks to your eating habits, your weight will land where it's supposed to be. Remember that each day might be different, but not vastly. By listening to your body, you'll become comfortable accommodating your carbohydrate needs.

Figuring out your carb tolerance is a process of trial and error. Start with a handful of carbs at each meal. If you find that you're gaining weight with this amount, try cutting it by half or taking the carbs out of one meal a day and choosing lower-carb snacks more often. It's a balance.

The key is knowing which carbs do what. There are three different classes of carbohydrate: starches, sugars, and cellulose, which is otherwise known as fiber and is found in fruits, vegetables, and grains.

STARCHES

When people hear the word "starch," they tend to imagine foods that are white, bland, and devoid of nutrition. But a lot of what we classify as starches are healthful, nutritious, whole foods that shouldn't be avoided. These include rice and any other grains, pasta, cereal, root vegetables, quinoa (which is a seed, FYI), oatmeal, and starchy vegetables such as corn, peas, potatoes, and winter squash.

STARCHY VEGETABLES

Let's start with starchy vegetables. I've heard one too many people describe starchy vegetables like potatoes and corn as junk, and that's just a shame. It's also not true, and referring to food in those terms—especially whole food that's straight from the earth—is not okay. What, are we supposed to feel bad about enjoying corn on the cob in August? Okay, well, more for me, then.

Starchy vegetables are a great way to get some carbs along with fiber and other nutrients, and there's no reason to stop enjoying them. They can increase your satiety during meals and give you lasting energy for all that you do. So please, stop avoiding them. When you do choose starchy vegetables at meals, just let them take the place of other carbs like rice or pasta. So, a handful at meals or a quarter of your plate.

GRAINS

When it comes to grains, there are two kinds: refined and whole.

Many whole grains have three parts: the endosperm, the bran, and the germ. The bran and the germ are full of fiber, antioxidants, vitamins, and minerals. When grains are refined, the nutritious bran and germ are removed, and we're left with the endosperm, which is basically what you're getting when you eat white flour, white rice, and the products made from them. Hello, soda crackers!

Another good example of a refined carb is hot wheat cereal. It contains wheat that has been stripped of its germ and bran, leaving a white, fiberless grain. On the other hand, lightly refined or unrefined carbs like whole wheat, steel-cut oats, and brown rice contain the entire grain and all of its nutrition.

The USDA recommends that at least half of our grain intake come from whole grains, which does leave a little wiggle room for those of you who can't stand brown rice or whole-wheat pasta. But you'll need to read food labels closely to see if you're really getting the whole grains you want. Watch out, though, because a product with the claim "made with whole grains" means its total grain content only has to be a minimum of 50 percent whole grain, which sometimes doesn't amount to a lot. Look for products with a "100 percent whole grains" claim on the packaging and check out the ingredients: Whole grains should be first or second.

THE DEAL WITH SUGAR CRASHES

The problem with consuming a lot of refined grains (or refined carbs in general) is that they're absorbed quicker by the body and can leave us with a "crash" in blood sugar. Here's how it goes: You eat a bag of sour candies or a big bowl of plain noodles for lunch. Because there's not a lot of fiber, fat, or protein in your meal, and the grains/sugars are refined, the glucose rushes into your blood very quickly. Your pancreas senses this and releases insulin to deal with your rising blood sugar. In people without diabetes, this rise in blood sugar will be fast, but still within normal glucose levels. The insulin rushes the glucose into your cells, and your blood sugar goes down. But in this case, because this all happens so quickly, you might feel like shit afterward. Your energy might drop. You might feel tired. You just ate, but you feel like you have no energy—this is a blood sugar crash. If you would have eaten a meal with high-fiber whole grains, plus some protein and fat, these nutrients would have slowed the release of sugar into your blood. Your blood glucose levels would have risen in a more moderate fashion, and the entire process would have taken more time. You would have felt energized and good after your meal.

For people who have diabetes or issues with blood sugar control, eating large portions of refined, ultraprocessed carbohydrates can cause higher blood sugar beyond normal glucose levels. This can be dangerous if it happens often or if glucose levels go too high. We can all mitigate these risks by eating fewer carbs, replacing refined carbs with less processed or whole ones, and eating them together with a protein and a fat to slow their absorption. Again, a rise in blood sugar after eating carbs is normal, but ideally this rise occurs slowly over time.

You may have heard of the Glycemic Index (GI), which is a ranking from 0–100—pure glucose being a score of 100—of how quickly certain carb-containing foods raise blood sugar after being eaten. Foods that are low on the Glycemic Index, such as peanuts (14) and kidney beans (27), cause a slow rise in blood sugar. On the other hand, foods that are high on the GI such as cornflakes (84) and white bread (70), raise blood sugar a lot quicker. The goal is to eat more foods that are low on the GI, which will help keep you feeling fuller for longer and, if you're diabetic, help with the control of blood sugars.

But the Glycemic Index is not so simple because we rarely eat foods in isolation. Sure, we eat peanuts on their own, but what about bagels (72 on the GI)? If we add fat, protein, or both to a bagel—maybe in the form of peanut butter, that will reduce the GI of the bagel because the fat and protein slow the release of the sugar from that bagel into the body. This also explains why peanut M&M's are low in the GI: They contain sugar, but they also have peanuts that contribute fat and protein. And fava beans? They sound healthy, but are high on the index (79) for whatever reason. A chocolate bar is a lot lower than that, at around a 49.

Other factors that can affect the Glycemic Index rank of a food include processing, type of carbohydrate, acid content, which slows carb metabolism, and if the food is cooked. The more a food is processed, the higher it tends to be because of the destruction of fibers—so whole fruit would be lower than a blended fruit smoothie. A baked potato has a GI of 85, but if you cook that baked potato and cool it, the GI is lower, because of the type of starch it contains. Cooked pasta has a GI of around 50, but if it's cooked to al dente, its Glycemic Index rank is lower. Adding a protein to your pasta will lower the GI even more.

Needless to say, while more nourishing foods tend to be low on the GI, using the GI as your sole tool to determine if a food is nutritious isn't really a good idea. The index is merely informational in terms of blood glucose, not actual nutrition.

BREAD

A lot of us have lost the joy in eating bread because we've been scared off it by the diet industry. We're told that bread is refined, gluten-containing junk that will do nothing but pack on the pounds. Obviously, this isn't true: Not all bread is highly refined, and eating carbs doesn't automatically make us gain weight unless—like any other food—we're eating too much of them.

The truth is that bread can be full of whole grains that provide fiber, protein, antioxidants, and vitamins. Whole grains like the ones in a less-refined bread also give us slow-burning energy. Above all else, a lot of us really like bread, and taking it out of our diets altogether feels restrictive and punishing.

When it comes to breads, it pays to know how to pick 'em. I usually have a heartier, nourishing Ezekiel bread for every day, but if you think I'm going to eat a hamburger or a BLT on anything but a super-refined white bread, you're sadly mistaken. And standing in my kitchen, eating sweet challah warm from the oven, with salted butter, is a memory I'll think of on my deathbed. I don't do it every day, but when it happens once in a while, it's fine. Just make sure your everyday bread is something wholesome and leave the sweet challah/baguette types for the other half of your grain intake—that's a more healthful way to enjoy breads.

Choosing a nourishing bread is simple. Remember, what you want to look for is 100 percent whole grain, not just "made with whole grains." Watch out for "multigrain"—that just means that the bread has several grains in it. Big deal. Similarly, brown bread may be white bread with molasses in it to give it a brown color. So sneaky! In other words, "brown" bread does not mean 100 percent whole grain. If you compare the labels between white bread and brown, there's seldom a difference. So don't automatically think that any bread that's brown or multigrain has more nutrition in it. Here are some other guidelines:

- You want something that has as little sugar in it as possible, preferably 0 grams. Most breads have a couple of grams per slice, so just try to go as low as possible.
- Grams of fiber per slice should be 2–3+.
- Sprouted grain breads are whole grain, and they generally have higher amounts of vitamins C and E, folate, and fiber.
- Breads that have 100 percent whole wheat contain all parts of the wheat, which bumps up the nutrition from antioxidants, fiber, vitamins, and minerals.
- If you're looking for a crisp bread or cracker, a Ryvita type with whole grains is perfect.

CEREALS

I'm not a huge fan of cold cereals in general because most of them are low in protein, highly refined, and sugary, leaving you starving about eight minutes after you eat them. Even cereals that contain manufactured protein or soy flakes just don't seem to satiate like such high-protein breakfast picks as eggs, a tofu scramble, or some ricotta on toast.

And as far as the "made with whole grains" claim, cereals are some of the worst offenders for using those words to give the product a health halo. Perfect example: Even though Lucky Charms claims to be made with whole grains, these are in small amounts and have been refined to death, resulting in a cereal still extremely low in fiber and full of sugar, FYI.

If cold cereal is something you don't want to give up, I'd recommend switching to a hearty type, such as muesli, and eating it with some Greek yogurt, just to bump up the protein. Look at the nutrition facts label for fiber grams (a cereal should ideally have around 5 grams of fiber per serving), check out the ingredients to see that whole grains are first on the list, and above all else, use your common sense. Oatmeal and other whole-grain cereals are a fantastic vehicle for fruit, nuts, and nut butters, and can be a higher-protein breakfast if you cook them in milk. Cooking oatmeal in chicken broth and serving it with scallions and a fried egg is also a delish way to create a savory breakfast.

SUGARS

Now that we've covered starches, let's move on to the second group of carbohydrates: sugars. Sugar can be naturally present in foods, and it can be added. Foods that contain natural sugars include fruit (fructose), dairy (lactose), and some vegetables such as corn and beets (sucrose). Added sugars are put into foods to make them sweet or sweeter. As you can imagine, there's a distinct nutritional difference between these two types.

I'm not here to tell you that added sugar is healthy or that you should be eating a lot of it. In general, we all should reduce our sugar intake, but there's no reason to cut sugar out of your life altogether. Doing that is not only close to impossible, it's miserable as hell.

Let's cut to the quick. Sugar is not toxic. Like gluten, people love to blame sugar for everything that's wrong in the world, but that's an extremely narrow-minded approach. Sure, as a population, we tend to eat too much added sugar, and yes—sugar, especially added sugar, is probably inflammatory. It's also an easy source of calories that has been linked to obesity, premature aging, cardiovascular disease, and negative effects on our gut bacteria.

But keep in mind that the standard American diet is typically high in fat and refined carbs, and low in fiber, so in research studies on people who are eating this diet, it's tough to separate the health effects that sugar may be having from other confounding factors in their diets and lifestyles. In other words, people who eat more sugar tend to have less nutrient-dense, more refined diets, which can have a huge impact on their overall health. Sugar isn't the only thing wrong with how many of us are eating, and to say that all of our health problems will be solved if we just cut sugar out of our diets isn't true. Nobody eats sugar in isolation; we're eating it with other things, for different reasons. We have to look at the whole picture. Read on.

NATURAL SUGARS

Natural sugars in fruit, dairy, and some vegetables are present alongside other nutrients such as fiber, antioxidants, vitamins, and minerals. The fiber in fruit and vegetables and the protein in dairy help our bodies absorb the natural sugars in these foods slower, which helps keep our blood sugar stable. So, to say that a piece of fruit is equal to candy is completely preposterous and misleading, yet I've seen this statement made plenty of times in the diet industry. The benefits of fruit far outweigh anything you'd get from a piece of candy, so please don't fall for this.

Can you eat too much natural sugar? Sure. Don't be like my dad, who used to sit down with a huge bowl of grapes and eat the entire thing. Oh, Dad. Too much of any sugar can cause elevated triglycerides, which are a type of fat that floats around in your blood and is used for energy, and an excess of energy will be stored as fat. Having high levels of triglycerides is associated with an increased risk for heart disease. That doesn't mean you should be avoiding foods that contain natural sugar. Just don't treat them like a free-for-all, which is true for almost anything we eat.

ADDED SUGARS

This is the part where we talk about desserts because obviously they're a source of added sugars in most of our diets. As I said above, there's nothing wrong with enjoying desserts and other sweet foods, but my recommendation is to be mindful of how much of your diet comes from them. A dessert a day? Okay. Two or three every day? Maybe not.

Unlike a lot of books that address eating, I'm not going to tell you that conventional desserts are bad and should only be sweetened with dates or maple syrup and never (gasp) white sugar! Oh no! I see a lot of bloggers who don't do the science posting recipes using "natural" sugars like honey or coconut sugar as if they're healthier than refined white sugar. First, white sugar is "natural," too. It mostly comes from sugar beets or sugarcane, which are *plants*. Second, research shows that all sugars are basically the same to our bodies once they're metabolized. Agave, the darling of wellness bloggers, is actually higher in fructose than high-fructose corn syrup, and it's still sugar, so don't be fooled. Your body doesn't care if you make brownies with raw cane sugar; it's still going to see it for what it is: sugar. Now, dates can be used as a sweetener, but they also contain fiber and nutrients, which add more value in terms of nutrition.

Apart from desserts, added sugars are mostly present in ultra-processed foods like candy, pastries, sugar-sweetened beverages, and are even in sneaky places like jarred spaghetti sauce and salad dressings. There are around sixty-one different names for sugar on food labels. Many will be obvious, like brown sugar or cane sugar, or even buttered syrup or high-fructose corn syrup—the words "sugar" and "syrup" give them away. Others are better disguised, such as barley malt, molasses, and the very virtuous-sounding brown rice syrup. (Brown rice! Healthy!)

the many names of sugar

If you see any of these names on a label, it's sugar:

Agave nectar	Glucose solids
Cane juice	Honey
Cane juice crystals	Maltodextrin
Caramel	Maltol
Corn sweetener	Maltose
Dehydrated cane juice	Mannose
Dextrin	Muscovado
Dextrose	Panocha
Evaporated cane juice	Saccharose
Fructose	Sucrose
Fruit juice	Sweet sorghum
Fruit juice concentrate	Treacle
Glucose	

Because nutrition labels are based on 100 grams of sugar in a 2,000-calorie diet, anything more than 15 percent of your daily value—which is 15 grams—is considered to be high in sugar. In the United States, labels have an added sugar line, which denotes the amount of nonnaturally occurring sugar in the product. This makes it a lot easier to compare the added sugars in different products and make a smarter choice in terms of which product to buy so you don't unknowingly add lots of sugar into your diet.

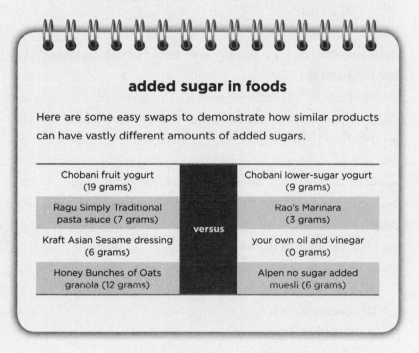

added sugar in foods

Here are some easy swaps to demonstrate how similar products can have vastly different amounts of added sugars.

	versus	
Chobani fruit yogurt (19 grams)		Chobani lower-sugar yogurt (9 grams)
Ragu Simply Traditional pasta sauce (7 grams)		Rao's Marinara (3 grams)
Kraft Asian Sesame dressing (6 grams)		your own oil and vinegar (0 grams)
Honey Bunches of Oats granola (12 grams)		Alpen no sugar added muesli (6 grams)

So, how much sugar should you be eating? The World Health Organization (WHO) recommends that adults and children consume fewer than 50 grams of sugars per day and that amount includes both added and natural sugars. Because I don't expect people to count grams of anything, I always recommend eating as little added sugar as possible. Some days you'll have more than others, but remember that the whole idea is to reduce your sugar intake to less than what it is now.

Teach your body to expect less sweet by slowly decreasing the amount of sugar you put into your food, and be aware of hidden sources of added sugars. As far as sweeteners go, use them if you like, but again: Use as little as possible. The goal is to decrease your sweet tolerance overall.

CELLULOSE

Cellulose, or fiber, is the third type of carbohydrate, and one of the most important.

Fiber can be soluble or insoluble—both types are not digestible and pass through the body. Sources of soluble fiber include legumes, oats, flaxseed, some fruits and vegetables such as sweet potatoes, brussels sprouts, strawberries, and oranges, and they nourish gut bacteria. Sources of insoluble fiber include whole grains, brans, and nuts and seeds, as well as fruits and vegetables with seeds and skins.

Here are some of the wonderful things fiber does:

- Lowers risk of cardiovascular disease
- Lowers cholesterol
- Keeps blood sugars stable
- Helps with regularity
- Feeds our gut bacteria
- May help keep you fuller, longer

We need around 25–38 grams of fiber a day. While fiber supplements can be high in sugar, they lack the nutrients that food provides, so I always suggest to clients that they get their fiber—and everything else—from food, not supplements. You certainly don't have to count grams of fiber, just eat more plants every day to increase your intake effortlessly!

CARB CRAVINGS

I hope you see by now that there is nothing inherently wrong with carbohydrate. It's a nutrient just like all other nutrients. It may be easier to overeat than fat or protein, but this isn't a good reason to take it out of your diet. Part of managing your intake is being aware of your cravings. Yes, carb cravings are a real thing. If you're having a lot of them, see if one of the following reasons may be the cause.

FATIGUE

When you're tired, your body is looking for quick energy, and carbs are that—especially sweet carbs like pastries. When you don't sleep well or enough, your body releases more ghrelin (remember the hunger hormone?), increasing your drive to eat. At the same time, leptin (the "stop eating" hormone) levels decrease, leading you to eat more. You may also have a spike in cortisol, which will also stimulate an appetite, especially for carbs. So let's just say it's three against one here, and you know who is probably going to win.

It's easy for me to tell you to just get more sleep, but as a mother and someone with an otherwise stressful life, I know that it's sometimes easier said than done. And there's nothing more obnoxious than people telling you to get more sleep, as if you wouldn't if it was in any way possible. What I'm going tell you is this: Make sure you have good sleep hygiene, because that can have a big impact on your weight and health. That means, no screens an hour before bed. Going to bed at a decent hour. Wearing earplugs to drown out your partner's snoring. You'll still hear the kids cry for you, trust me on that one. I've been wearing earplugs faithfully for the past couple of decades. No kidding. I'm serious about my sleep.

HORMONES

Ladies, having some carb cravings around that time of the month? There's the little issue of serotonin around your period. Serotonin is a hormone that's responsible in part for our mood and feelings of well-being. During the time before your period, serotonin levels drop, sometimes making you feel like crap. And because serotonin is made from carbs, guess what you're going to crave? So know that you may want some carbs at these times and have some more nourishing options available, such as 100 percent whole-grain bread, potatoes, and brown rice. Increase your protein and water intake to keep you satiated and hydrated, too.

STRESS

Just like when we're not sleeping well, being under stress messes with our hypothalamic pituitary adrenal axis, otherwise known as the HPA axis. The HPA axis manages our stress response by triggering the release of neurotransmitters like epinephrine and norepinephrine.[1] Our bodies react to these substances with the fight or flight response.

Humans first used our fight or flight response when we were cave dwellers and a feral tiger or mammoth was chasing us. Our bodies would basically drop everything and serve our immediate need for energy. The stress of encountering something that wants to gobble you up is a lot of work, after all. Your heart pounds, your breathing rate increases, and a whole host of other things happen in preparation for helping you survive.

Even though we don't have any brontosaurus giving us side-eye nowadays, our fight or flight response is triggered by everyday stress: overworking, getting every sickness the kids bring home from day care, pulling all-nighters to study . . . hey, life happens.

Among other things, fight or flight increases our cortisol levels, which tells the body to release glucose and fat from the muscles and liver to give our body the energy it needs to deal with the stressor. But once that glucose is used up and our blood sugar drops, we crave carbs. Because sugary, more refined carbs such as ice cream and chips are the fastest sources of glucose, we usually reach for those. These elevate our blood sugar and curb our cravings for a while but can result in quite the blood sugar crash, which can lead to fatigue and then more carb cravings. Are you getting dizzy yet? It's quite the vicious cycle, and it can have a detrimental effect on our health.

So what's the answer? First of all, try to alleviate at least some of the stress in your life. Sheesh, stop overloading yourself already! Nobody ever said to themselves, "Am I ever sad that I stopped being the class parent!" or "I'm so glad that I went to every single PTA meeting; those were just SO memorable!" Say no to anything that's not mandatory, and let go of whatever you can in your schedule. Taking time for yourself isn't optional, so please do it.

Second, we all know that stress is as inevitable as death and taxes, so when it strikes, try to feed carb cravings with whole grains, starchy vegetables, and legumes. Their fiber content can help stabilize blood sugar instead of spiking and crashing it, and they're more nutritious than ultraprocessed food.

COMFORT

Carbs are also frequently associated with comfort food, which we crave when we're stressed. And like we discussed earlier, sometimes when we're upset, we turn to food to comfort us. It usually doesn't help us feel better in the long run, but it happens. Instead of immediately reaching for something to eat, take a moment to understand what you're feeling. Sit with those feelings for a bit and work through them. Is there anything you can do to alleviate your stress that doesn't involve food? If you still want to eat in response to your stress, go ahead, and then move on.

LOW-CARB INTAKE

Not eating enough carbs can cause you to crave them. If this is the case, you may need to increase your carbs a bit. Nutrition is trial and error, so if you feel as though you need to eat more carbs, add another spoonful or handful to your meals, or include a carb in your snacks.

LOW-CARB DIETS

This chapter wouldn't be complete if I didn't include a section on low-carb diets. Low carb, which I consider anything below 150 grams of carbs a day, doesn't have to mean keto, which is around 20–50 grams of carbs a day, depending on the person. There's a whole range of carb levels that someone can choose from without going to either end of the spectrum.

When people ask me what I think of low-carb eating plans, I think they expect me to be fully against that way of eating. I'm actually not, because for some people, eating very few carbs works. And for many of us, it doesn't. Let me explain.

Keto is by far the most popular diet out there right now that involves carb-controlling. You'll find a lot of people online and in real life who say that keto is super easy and they feel euphoric and "Oh my god, they've lost so much weight on it." The goal of the ketogenic diet is to be in ketosis, which is the physiological process when a scarcity of carbohydrates forces the body to burn stored fat for energy. It usually takes up to a week of eating less than 50 grams of carbs a day to achieve nutritional ketosis.

Many people think that keto is a high-protein diet, but it's not. In fact, eating too much protein can kick you out of ketosis. The keto diet is low in carbs (around 5 percent), moderate in protein (around 15 percent), and high in fat (around 70–80 percent). To stay in ketosis and burn fat, you have to eat a lot of fat, which can be hard to do. Some people resort to eating much of that fat in saturated form, which may be harmful to their health, as we'll discuss later. A keto diet can be followed in a healthier manner, but that still doesn't include a free-for-all of bacon and cheese. More like, green vegetables, avocado, and fish, for healthier balance of fats, along with fiber.

Still, keto works for some, but many people have trouble sustaining the diet because of what they can't eat. It's hard to give up most fruits, grains, birthday cake, fresh warm croissants, and your nonna's lasagna, but they are forbidden or strictly limited on keto. And if you break ketosis, the diet stops working. Unlike many other diets, you can't break keto and then just get back on it a million times—it only works when you're in ketosis. You need to stay true to the cause, and that's tough, especially because there's an emotional component to food that adds positive experiences to our lives. All in all, a low-carb or ketogenic diet is not the holy grail of weight loss. Research shows that neither of those eating plans is more effective for weight loss than a low-fat diet.[2]

Going too low in carbs isn't fun. You might find that you're sluggish, you have less endurance and tolerance for exercise, your mood may suffer, and you likely won't feel satisfied at meals. You might notice that you're more anxious because when the body doesn't get enough carbs, cortisol levels increase and send a signal to your central stress response system to wind down on pituitary-gland hormone production.[3] Unfortunately, the pituitary gland makes thyroid and other hormones that can affect your periods, mood, energy, blood sugar, body temperature, heart rate, blood pressure, sex drive, and more. So when it goes down, you do, too. In other words, there's a good chance that low-carb eating will make you feel like shit because you're eating too few carbs and your body doesn't like it.

There is no advantage to beating up your body and feeling like crap. Even if you do lose weight—which will be tough because of your elevated cortisol—is it really worth it? No. No, it's not. There's another way: by learning to manage your intake without crazy restrictions.

THE TRUTH ABOUT GLUTEN

A lot of pseudoscientific diets and the people who develop them like to pontificate to anyone who will listen that gluten is poison. They say it's responsible for cancer, ADHD, rashes, autoimmune disease, autism, depression, brain fog, global warming, plagues of locusts, and the low-rise jean trend. Unless you're suffering from a medical condition that causes you to not be able to eat gluten-containing grains, there are zero reasons to give them up. In fact, there are millions of people who eat gluten-free diets unnecessarily, which boggles my mind.

There is nothing beneficial about eating a grain-free diet.

Grain-free diets like Paleo like to say that early humans never ate grains, which is false. Actually, they ate whatever they could scrounge up because that was life in the Paleo era. Paleolithic humans were also a lot more active than we are: their average life expectancy was around thirty-five and their genetics were different. Their lives were in so many ways completely different from ours are now.

I see a lot of people trying to justify certain extreme diets by saying that certain civilizations ate X diet and lived healthy lives. The problem with this sort of comparison—besides the fact that it's usually overblown and untrue—is we have different lifestyles, genetics, and access to food than other ethnic groups living in other eras and/or parts of the world. Many of those groups actually weren't as physically healthy as we make them out to be. Their lives may have been shorter and far more challenging. Regardless, it's a red flag for me when I see someone making a comparison of this sort.

Sometimes, people react to gluten-containing foods with bloating, gas, diarrhea, and abdominal discomfort. They blame gluten for these symptoms, but recent research shows that in fact, gluten might be an innocent party. The guilt may lie squarely with fructans, a type of fermentable carbohydrate. Foods that are high in fructans are any wheat-containing foods, garlic, onions, cabbage, broccoli, and asparagus. Wheat and onions contribute 95 percent of the fructans in our diet, which is why when someone who is intolerant to fructans goes on a gluten-free diet, they usually see a resolution in their symptoms. But that's because they're cutting out fructans, not gluten. Insulin, which is naturally present in the above food and also added to foods to increase their fiber content, is a fructan and can easily be spotted on food labels.

If you suspect that you might be gluten- or fructan-intolerant, make sure you don't just blindly cut foods out of your diet in a bid to alleviate your symptoms. That's like shooting into darkness. It's always better to go see someone who has experience in these conditions, such as an RD or an allergist MD.

myth buster:

lectins are toxic.

You may have heard about lectins, which are sort of like the new gluten. Certain diets that I won't mention here have recently popularized the fear of lectins and give us something else to worry about unnecessarily. Lectins are a class of proteins called antinutrients, found in about 30 percent of the foods we eat, including grains. Proponents of grain-, nightshade-, and legume-free diets claim that these proteins are toxic and are responsible for health issues such as inflammation and all sorts of chronic diseases.

Chickpeas, one of the lectin-containing foods that many people avoid, were one of the first cultivated crops on earth. Don't you think that we'd have stopped eating them by now if they were so toxic? I mean, we've had since 3200 BC to figure it out. Also, North Americans don't happen to eat a lot of lectin-containing foods: Most of us are low in vegetables and legumes, so how is it that lectins are causing so much disease? Hint: they're not. Most of us can eat lectins without any deleterious effects.

While it's true that lectins are made by plants as a protective mechanism and that some are more toxic than others, humans have evolved to have the enzymes that break lectins down. We also cook the most toxic lectins—like the ones in kidney beans—which destroys the structure of those proteins, rendering them harmless. Some people have dysfunctional enzymes that don't properly break down lectins, leading to gut and autoimmune issues. But even in these cases, you might not need to cut out all lectin-containing foods. An elimination diet can help determine which foods are causing you problems and which ones aren't. Again, if you are lectin-intolerant you'll want to speak to an RD who is qualified to direct you on what the next steps are for this.

THE THEORY OF CARBOHYDRATE-INSULIN

Some people theorize that high insulin levels brought on by carb-rich diets facilitate fat storage and make it hard to lose weight. They believe that low-carb diets lower insulin levels, therefore allowing the body to release fat for burning. This is called the carbohydrate-insulin model of obesity.[4]

Yes, starches and sugars make our blood sugars rise; cellulose doesn't. But that's not a bad thing: Blood sugar is supposed to rise when we fuel our bodies. That's a normal physiological reaction. In people with diabetes or who have blood sugar issues, it's also okay to have a small bump in blood sugars after eating; we just don't want blood sugar to rise too quickly or too high. Eating whole grains and less refined carbs with sources of protein and fat will help stabilize blood sugar.

While a low-carb diet has been shown to decrease insulin levels, whether you'll burn more fat on that diet, especially compared to a low-fat diet, is controversial, and so is the carb-insulin model.[5] None of that matters, of course, if you follow an eating plan that's unsustainable and makes your life difficult and sad. There's a happy medium between high and low carb. Find yours.

Some people can tolerate lower carbs than others. And some people, like me for example, run on carbs. The secret is not to go crazy with carbs, but also not to go too low. The other secret is not to go on a low-carb diet just because somebody told you that carbs are horrible for you. Hopefully by now you know that they're not, and anyone who paints an entire food group with a uniformly shitty brush doesn't deserve the time of day anyhow. The research about low-carb diets and weight loss isn't very supportive in terms of them having any advantage over other types of eating plans. The best diet is what you can sustain.

Remember that no foods are off-limits, so if you love your potatoes and your bread, you can definitely have them. This is about normalizing all foods and getting rid of those "do not eat" lists that you've been storing in your head for far too long. It's also about you telling me what works for you, not the other way around. Only you know your body.

And while I'm not going to (and can't) give you an exact-grams-of-carbohydrate number to shoot for, you'll find your best level by trial and error. Sometimes you might need more, sometimes less. But remember: You want a diet that allows you to eat what you love. That makes you feel satisfied, physically and emotionally. That is free of guilt. That isn't a *diet*.

prioritize protein

Unlike carbs, protein's star has risen exponentially in the past few years. It's the darling of the food industry as well as diet culture. I think it's pretty unfair that protein gets all of the adoration while carbs are sent to the time-out corner. All in all, our love affair with protein is sort of warranted, but maybe a bit overblown at times. We need protein, but putting it into everything has become something of a marketing trick.

Protein is a multitasker if I've ever seen one. Not only does it provide vital nourishment, it's also a big part of ensuring we feel fuller, longer after eating. And it's tasty! I'm talking steaks, tofu, *bacon*, and chickpeas. Protein, both plant and animal, is a valuable nutrient.

When it comes to weight loss and maintaining weight, you may have heard that eating a lot of protein can help make and keep you lean. This is probably why companies are putting protein into everything now, including granola bars, water, and vodka. Okay, maybe not vodka . . . yet. That's totally happening, though.

Research does indeed suggest that people who eat more protein—and note that I'm not saying fewer carbs, I'm just saying more protein, calories being equal in both instances—tend to lose more weight than their lower-protein counterparts.[1] This is probably because protein is the toughest macronutrient for the body to break down. Carbs are pretty easy, because they're essentially turned into sugar. Fat is, well, fat. But protein is a whole other story.

Most of us get enough protein without even trying, even vegans, many of whom dread having to once again answer the question "But how do you get enough protein?" (Stop asking it.) But there are some things you need to know, like how much we really need at meals; how timing affects how protein can benefit us; how protein can help with appetite, weight loss, and maintenance; and yes: how vegans can get enough protein. This chapter will break down the ins and outs of this superstar macronutrient.

WHAT IS PROTEIN?

Protein, as we know it, is chains of amino acids that are present in food. During digestion, these amino-acid chains are broken down into individual amino acids by our digestive enzymes. The liver then reassembles these amino acids into different chains, to suit whichever process or area of the body they're needed in, and sends them on their way.

Protein is like the cinder block of macronutrients: It's the structure that holds up the house. Aside from making up most of our hair, nails, organs, and muscles, it's also a part of our DNA, bones, skin, blood, and other fluids. It's essential for the production of hormones, enzymes, antibodies, and cells. Unlike carbohydrate or fat, our body has no way of storing protein in its current form. Any extra-dietary protein that's not used immediately by our body is broken down and stored as triglycerides in fat cells or excreted as nitrogen in the urine.

We'd be lost without protein. The body can even convert protein into glucose and ketones in a process called catabolysis if it absolutely needs energy, and carbs and fat aren't available. This only happens in dire situations like starvation, and the source of this protein is usually muscle tissue. Not ideal, but then neither is death, and protein is working hard to avoid that. Not getting enough protein can cause problems such as the muscle breakdown, slow muscle recovery, low energy, lowered immunity, thinning hair and nails, dry skin, and nutrient malabsorption. That being said, it's pretty rare for someone, even vegans and vegetarians, to inadvertently have a protein deficiency because protein can be found in so many of our favorite foods.

Proteins come from either animal or plant sources. You probably know that beef, chicken, turkey, eggs, and fish are basically all protein. Plant-based proteins include tofu, tempeh, seitan, legumes, natto (fermented soybeans), nuts, hemp hearts, and seeds. Other foods such as dairy, grains, and some vegetables also contain protein. We'll get into the nitty-gritty of what each of these types of protein offers later on in the chapter.

Proteins are categorized as either being "complete" or "incomplete." There are twenty amino acids, and a complete protein is one that has all twenty.[2, 3] Your body needs all twenty of these to function. Our incredible body can actually make some of those amino acids on its own. Nine others are what we call "essential," meaning that we need to get them from our diet. And then there are conditional amino acids, which we can make when we're healthy, but not when we're stressed or ill. In those cases, we need to get them in food or supplements.

Most animal sources of protein, including cow's milk, and soy are complete. Plant-sourced proteins are usually incomplete, with one or two missing amino acids (what we dietitians call a "limiting" amino acid).

But most of us don't make a point of eating one type of protein day in and day out, and even with a limited diet, amino acids are found in enough foods that getting all twenty isn't really a problem. We used to recommend that incomplete proteins like beans, nuts, and grains be consumed together with complementary proteins to "make up" and "complete" them. Beans and rice were a favorite—beans supply the amino acids that the rice doesn't have, and the other way around. Now we know that as long as a person eats a balanced diet throughout the day that's rich in various proteins, their body will complete the proteins itself. No need to eat complementary proteins at the same meal.

PROTEIN AND WEIGHT LOSS

Other than, you know, keeping us alive, why are amino acids so important? Well, they're one of the reasons why protein can help with weight loss. Disassembling all of those amino-acid chains and reassembling them into what our body needs—which is what happens when we eat protein—is a lot of work. So, it takes our body more energy to digest protein than it does to digest carbs or fats. In fact, we burn 20–30 percent of the protein calories we eat just by messing with amino acids. In other words, the Thermic Effect of Food (TEF)—or the energy it takes to digest what we eat—is much higher for protein than carbs (5–10 percent) and fat (0–3 percent).[4]

The other reason? Protein plays a huge role in the satiety of your meals.[5] Think about a time when you had cold cereal for breakfast versus a time when you had eggs. What filled you up faster and for longer? I'm betting it was the eggs, because eggs are pure protein, and protein is filling because of what it does to your hormones. The consumption of protein triggers a decrease in ghrelin (that hunger hormone) and an increase in PYY, cholecystokinin, and GLP-1. All you need to know about those last three hormones is that they are anorexigenic, meaning they make us feel full, and they get going whenever we eat. A high-protein meal elicits a greater response from them compared to a high-carb meal.[6,7]

If you're looking to lose some weight, I often recommend replacing some carbs with protein because it does tend to result in a caloric deficit from satiety, TEF, and who knows what else.[8] Carbs are easy to overeat. Protein, not so much. There is the Protein Leverage Theory, which suggests that our bodies are biologically driven to consume adequate protein.[9] When we eat a carb-heavy, low-protein diet, our body senses it, and we experience a drive to overeat until we can glean enough protein from our food. Although more information is needed to prove this outright, it would explain a lot about how carbs are so easy to overconsume and why we don't seem to have an off switch when our protein intake is low.

Of course, this doesn't mean that if you want to lose weight (or not), you should forsake all other macronutrients and turn into a carnivore dieter, eating only meat, salt, and water. Protein foods aren't a free-for-all. Protein is a macronutrient like fat and carbs, and as with the others, if you eat too much of it, you'll gain weight. What it does mean is that all of your meals should have adequate protein. I see a lot of people who eat salads with a few tablespoons of nuts as a protein for lunch, and they're hungry an hour later. Or they have a bagel with butter, cereal, or toast with jam for breakfast. Then they're foraging for something else to eat long before lunch.

I love bagels, but eating a meal without a significant amount of protein is just not likely to keep you full for very long.

GUIDELINES FOR PROTEIN INTAKE

Protein requirements depend on your size, your sex, how active you are, and what your goals are. Are you a serious bodybuilder? Are you sedentary? Do you do some sort of strenuous activity several times a week?

Okay, we're going to do some math here, but I promise, it'll be painless. For years and years, the FDA standard protein recommendation has been between 0.8–1.0 grams per kilogram, which is 54–68 grams a day for a 150-pound person. But we now know that this amount may be too little, especially for people who are older, active, pregnant, or nursing. Science shows that most healthy, moderately active adults need around 1.2 grams of protein per kilogram, which comes out to around 82 grams for a 150-pound person. That's a huge difference from what we previously were recommending! And if you're an athlete, you'll probably need even more. For more personalized recommendations, see a sports RD.

In general, most healthy people benefit from eating around 20–25 grams of protein per meal. That's for satiety, muscle building, and energy. The good news? Most of us get enough protein without counting and managing grams per day, so don't think about that math too much. Instead, I want to you to visualize what 20–25 grams of protein looks like, so you know going into your meal how filling some chicken is going to be versus an egg. And although some of the plant-based proteins don't add up as fast, you can cobble a couple together to make it to that 20 grams (because 2 cups of beans, no thank you).

Here's what the USDA says:

Food	Portion	Protein
Tempeh	6 oz.	33 grams
Chicken (cooked)	3.5 oz.	29 grams
Beef (cooked)	3.5 oz.	28 grams
Salmon and most other fish (cooked)	3.5 oz.	25 grams
Shrimp (cooked)	3.5 oz.	24 grams
Tuna (canned)	5 oz.	27 grams
Tofu	½ cup	10 grams
Greek yogurt	3.5 oz.	9 grams
Lentils (canned)	½ cup	9 grams
Black beans (canned)	½ cup	8 grams
Chickpeas	½ cup	7 grams
Cheddar cheese	1 oz.	6 grams
Eggs	1 egg	6 grams
Ricotta	¼ cup	5 grams
Nuts	1 oz.	5 grams

Food is more than just numbers, and again, I don't want you to feel as though you have to count grams of anything. While protein is an important part of the equation, it's obviously not the only piece of the nutrition puzzle.

PROTEIN QUALITY

I talk a lot about protein quality with my clients, because understanding which proteins are high quality and which aren't can help them put together meals that are satisfying and nutritious.

There are several ways of measuring protein quality, namely the moderately confusing but official Protein Digestibility Corrected Amino Acid Score (PDCAAS), which is used by the FDA.[10] This system takes into account the amino-acid profile of each protein and its bioavailability to the body—in other words, how much of the protein our body can actually absorb and convert to make into other proteins.

Because drilling everything down to individual amino acids is both ambitious and sort of a waste of time for most people, I have my own system that's simple. Our goal is to get 20–25 grams of protein per meal. If a protein source can get you to that level in a portion that's not over-the-top, it's high quality.

Here's how I classify proteins:

- ✗ High-quality proteins can be used as primary sources. These include meat, fish, eggs, Greek yogurt, ricotta, tofu, tempeh, and beans.

- ✗ Moderate-quality proteins should be used as secondary, or adjunct, sources. These include cheese, nuts, nut butters, hemp hearts and other seeds, regular yogurt, and sprouted grain bread.

- ✗ Low-quality proteins are foods that contain protein, but in such small amounts that they definitely need to be boosted with other significant sources. These include most refined carbs and most protein-containing vegetables (e.g., broccoli has 2 grams per cup).

So, those two tablespoons of nuts on your salad might contribute 2 or 3 grams of protein, and sure, you can eat them with an ounce of cheese (6 grams) and maybe some croutons (1 gram), but you're not even coming close to 20 grams. On the other hand, if you throw ½ cup of black beans onto your salad, that will give you 8 grams of protein. Three and a half ounces of chicken breast will contribute around 29 grams. Two eggs have 12 grams. See what I mean? Unless you want to eat a cup of nuts and half a bar of cheese, you're probably better off using those moderate-quality proteins as adjuncts to higher-quality proteins.

The sprouted grain bread I eat has 7 grams of protein in two slices. Topped with two tablespoons of peanut butter, that gets me to 15 grams. But if I top my toast with 2 eggs, it gets me to 21 grams. A ¾ cup serving of normal yogurt with fruit has around 9 grams of protein. But if I swap it out for Greek yogurt and add a tablespoon of almonds, I've got around 20 grams. And ricotta? Such an underused protein. If I top my two slices of bread with ½ cup of ricotta, it gets really close to that 20-gram number at 17 grams.

PROTEIN AT EACH MEAL

When you eat your protein is just as important as what your source is. Historically, we've eaten a low-protein breakfast (think: pancakes, toast, waffles, cereal), a moderate-protein lunch (a sandwich with a few ounces of deli meat), and a protein-heavy dinner (meat and potatoes). Some research even shows that most of us can't absorb more than 35 grams at one time, although that number is contentious.

While you can certainly meet your protein requirements in this fashion, it's not the best way to do it. Our muscles need a continuous source of protein to help them build and repair themselves. And since we can't really store protein in our bodies, it's important to have protein gradually throughout the day:[11]

- ✕ 20–25 grams at breakfast
- ✕ 20–25 grams at lunch
- ✕ 20–25 grams at dinner
- ✕ 5–10 grams for snacks (combining protein with a fat and a carb will level up your snack to something that actually tides you over to your next meal)

Protein makes meals more filling, which helps prevent 2 p.m. food foraging expeditions in the office break room and it keeps us alert, which means you won't be locking yourself in your office to take a midmorning nap. (Yes, I did that when I was pregnant and all I could eat was carbs. And yes, someone did walk in on me while I was sleeping in the darkened room. So embarrassing.) The object of the game is to keep yourself awake, alert, and satiated while providing a steady stream of protein to your muscles.

Because different amino acids can be found across different proteins—both in animal and plant sources—variety of diet is important to our overall health, whether we're omnivores, vegetarians, or vegans. For omnivores, there really is room for all the proteins you love, including bacon, steak, and the occasional ballpark hot dog. The trick is to switch things up. For example, if you're used to eating a ton of meat, try a few plant-based meals every week by experimenting with tofu, lentils, or other vegan proteins.

PLANT-BASED DIETS

Plant-based diets are super trendy right now, and it's one trend I can get behind 100 percent. You may think "plant-based" means a vegetarian or vegan diet, but the definition varies from person to person. Some vegans and vegetarians use plant-based to describe their diet, but I believe that having a plant-based diet doesn't necessarily mean that you're eating only plants or that you're vegan. Plant-based diets can also be omnivorous, but with the majority of the diet being plants. I love the term "plant-forward," which perfectly describes a diet that has a large amount of plants, but also some animal foods. I personally eat what would be described as a plant-forward diet.

We'll talk more about plant-based diets in a later chapter, but to answer an age-old question that's unfortunately still being asked: yes. You can easily get enough protein whether or not you're consuming any animal products.

Read on to get the real deal on all proteins.

ANIMAL PROTEINS

RED MEAT

Somewhere in the 1980s, we got the impression that red meat is bad, and dry, poached chicken breast is good. That's simply not true and I'm not going to tell you to ditch the steak in favor of grilled chicken. Whether it's beef, pork, turkey, chicken, or fish, my philosophy is that it's all about portion size and frequency.

When it comes to red meat like beef, the thing to be aware of is that it generally has more saturated fat than white meat. Saturated fat has long been maligned as being horrible for our health and has been linked with cardiovascular disease, stroke, diabetes, inflammation, and a lot of other issues. We'll get into this in the next chapter, but for now, let me just say that it's about balance. As long as you're not eating an 18-oz. porterhouse every day, most healthy people can consume steak once or twice a week without an issue. Red meat has high levels of zinc, iron, and selenium, and is easy to prepare. It can also be extremely budget-friendly.

Grass-Fed Versus Grain-Fed Beef

If you're wondering whether you should be choosing grass-fed beef over grain-fed, I've got your answer. Grass-fed is generally leaner, with higher concentrations of omega-3 fatty acids and a fat called CLA, or conjugated linoleic acid, than grain-fed beef. Both are good for us, and proponents of grass-fed beef will try to impress its superiority on you. The problem is that even though grass-fed beef contains these beneficial fats, the amount that it actually has is super small. And how much beef are you really going to eat, anyhow?

My thought is that you're better off eating the beef you can afford (which is, for most people, not grass-fed), and looking elsewhere to boost your good-fat profile.

Grain-fed beef is often portrayed as coming from feedlots, where cows are stuffed into overcrowded pens and fed completely unnatural diets of genetically modified corn, but not all factory farms treat their animals poorly, in the same way that not all grass-fed cattle are frolicking around in a field of daisies, happy as can be. So while it's tempting and easy to draw these sorts of conclusions—grass-fed is idyllic and healthy, grain-fed is oppressive and unhealthy—it's not that simple.

WHITE MEATS

White meats include chicken, turkey, and pork. Chicken and turkey have historically had a health halo compared to red meat due to their lower levels of saturated fat, at least in their breast meat. But even the dark meat from poultry contains mostly unsaturated fats, along with a lot of nutrients such as zinc, iron, and selenium—all of which are necessary for good health. So if you prefer dark meat, but have been choosing white meat at Thanksgiving dinner, don't worry about it! Have that juicy chicken leg and enjoy it. As far as "the other white meat" goes, pork is known to be a fantastic source of B vitamins, and the lean cuts are low in saturated fats.

Again, it's the quality of your diet overall that matters—so mix up your protein sources.

FISH AND SEAFOOD

Fish and seafood are a delicious source of high-quality protein that a lot of people skip because they either don't like it, don't know how to cook it, or aren't in the habit of buying it—or it's too expensive. If you don't like fish, I don't think you need to choke it down just because it's healthy. The same goes for any food! If you're looking for the most cost-effective fish and seafood, unseasoned frozen varieties can be a lot less expensive than fresh ones.

But if you're not eating it because you have no idea how to cook it, it's worth learning. Many of my clients are afraid of overcooking their fish and making it rubbery. I wouldn't want that either, so here are a few cooking tips to help you out.

Fish has gotten a reputation for being healthy because of fish oils, which are omega-3 fatty acids otherwise known as DHA (docosahexaenoic acid) and EPA (eicosapentaenoic acid). In the 1990s, we believed that fish oil was beneficial for a wide range of health issues, especially heart disease. Dietitians were telling everyone to eat fatty fish three or more times a week, and companies started fortifying their eggs, orange juice, and breads with omega-3 fatty acids. It was like fish oil was the gold standard for heart health—and totally worth those fishy burps from taking supplements.

As of now, we're finding out that fish oils aren't as magical as we previously thought. They're not harmful, but the latest research suggests that while they appear to have a positive effect on memory and triglycerides, they don't appear to lower risk for cardiovascular disease.[12, 13, 14] For those with head injury, inflammation, depression, ADHD, cholesterol, blood sugars, and more, the research is mixed; some of these conditions appear to improve with very high doses of DHA, but only in specific individuals. All this means is that you might want to reconsider those fish-oil supplements.

But you definitely don't want to stop eating fish. Aside from being a high-quality protein, the EPA and DHA in fish and seafood do have some benefits such as helping to lower triglycerides. The best sources of EPA and DHA are fish and omega-3 eggs. If you're

how to cook fish and seafood

- ✖ Fish cooks at about eight minutes per inch of thickness.
- ✖ Fish and seafood continue to cook once they're removed from the heat source, so if your fish is slightly underdone, remove it from heat and let it stand for a couple minutes.
- ✖ Fillets less than half an inch don't have to be flipped.
- ✖ Thin, delicate fish like flounder or sole tends to overcook quickly, so avoid grilling it; it's best done in the oven or a pan on the stovetop.
- ✖ Cook shrimp with the shells on to prevent them from getting rubbery and add flavor to the dish.
- ✖ Seafood like shrimp and scallops cook very quickly, so watch them carefully.
- ✖ You can always broil fish, but one of my favorite ways to cook thicker, skin-on fillets is in a pan on the stovetop. Heat a neutral oil in a heavy pan until the oil shimmers and the pan is blazing hot, then lay the fish skin side down. Cook until the flesh is almost opaque, flip for a minute, then remove from the pan.
- ✖ Roasting fish fillets is simple! Use parchment paper or foil to line a pan, lay fillets on the pan, and place in preheated oven (350°F is fine). You can also make parchment or foil pouches with fish and veggies. Use vegetables that cook quickly, like green beans or spinach, and wrap with fillet, seasonings, and a pat of butter or olive oil.

Remember that you can always put something back into the oven if it needs it, but once you overcook it, you can't take it back.

a vegan, I recommend an omega-3 supplement made from micro-algae, which is a plant form of DHA and EPA.

Farmed Versus Wild Fish

Many believe that farmed fish is lesser quality than wild fish. While farmed fish in some areas has been shown to be environmentally unfriendly, it's not all bad. Some aquaculture is done with sustainable practices and has very little impact on the environment.

Wild fish is in the same boat. Anything caught wild has sort of a health halo around it, but in reality, that might not be the case. Some species are overfished. Some are caught using underpaid and forced labor. And some originate in waters that aren't necessarily the cleanest. Wild fish is usually a lot more expensive than farmed, which puts it out of reach for a large number of people who would otherwise consume fish.

Whether you choose farmed or wild, you can read more about your choice and its sustainability on the Monterey Bay Aquarium Seafood Watch website.[15]

In general, all animal protein—beef, pork, poultry, and fish—when raised for food, creates environmental complications such as water and farmland use and greenhouse gas production.[16] But so do plant proteins, perhaps to a lesser extent. So we do need to be cognizant of these things and take them into account when planning our meals. I'm not saying to never eat meat, but to eat it less often, with plant-based meals interspersed throughout the week.

EGGS

Eggs are inexpensive little bombs of pure, high-quality protein. Yes, even the yolks, which contain lutein and zeaxanthin—carotenoids that are important for eye health—and choline, an important nutrient that's essential for liver, muscle, brain, nervous system, and cell health.[17,18] The yolks also have all of the fat in eggs. Without fat, your meal won't be as satiating, and hey—the nineties called. They want their egg-white omelets back. You can add fat with avocados and cheese, but still, the yolks are healthy. So please, don't ditch them.

We used to believe that eggs could influence blood cholesterol and the risk of cardiovascular disease because of their high cholesterol content. But science says the opposite: Dietary cholesterol does not significantly affect blood cholesterol in most healthy people.[19] Most people can eat eggs every day, yolks included, without having to worry about anything.

PLANT PROTEINS

Let's clear this up once and for all: Just because someone doesn't eat animals doesn't mean they're automatically deficient in protein. Our bodies absorb plant-based proteins comparatively well compared to animal proteins, provided that over the course of the day, we're eating a variety of plant proteins that complete each other.[20]

Some examples of plant proteins are lentils, beans, tofu, and tempeh. Plant proteins are versatile, budget-friendly, and nourishing, and the consensus among scientists is that the general population doesn't eat nearly enough of them. While most vegan proteins also contain carbohydrate, they're still a healthful way to get your protein. Unfortunately, many in our carb-phobic society will turn their backs on plant proteins because they can't see how their "good proteins" outweigh their "bad carbs." But you know better, right?

There's a huge push right now for meat-alternative burgers, crumbles—like meatless ground beef—and sausages. While these products are ultraprocessed, they're a reasonable alternative to their meat-based counterparts for those of you who don't eat meat. But

I wouldn't say that these products are healthier for our bodies than meat because they're still very refined, so if you do eat meat, don't go ordering a fully loaded meatless burger thinking it's a much better choice healthwise. In most cases, it's not.

SOY

The majority of soy foods—tofu, tempeh, protein powder, and soy milk—are made by processing soybeans from the soybean plant. Soybeans themselves are often eaten whole and roasted, or steamed in the pod. I love soy as a protein source because it's nutrient-dense, it's inexpensive, and it's easy to prepare. It's also a complete protein and contains fiber, B vitamins, and antioxidants such as isoflavones.

Tofu is one of my fav soy foods because it's inexpensive, and it subs in for meat in almost any dish. For instance, I do butter tofu instead of butter chicken, I use tofu in Asian lettuce wraps instead of ground pork, and I scramble it instead of eggs. I also love to coat tofu in batter and panfry it. Delish.

Tempeh, which is fermented soy, is a bit scary at first when you pick it up at the store. It's sort of lumpy and hard, and it's tough to imagine what you can actually do with a brick of it. But not only is tempeh nutty and delicious, it's filling AF. You can use it as a bacon substitute, or bake it with teriyaki or peanut sauce. It's also a great meat substitute in sandwiches, stir-fries, and even dumplings.

For snacks and in bowl meals, edamame are high-protein perfection. I buy them frozen and steam them, then sprinkle with salt. My kids love them, too.

myth buster:

soy causes diseases.

Soy has gotten a bit of a bad rap lately. Some men are afraid to eat soy protein because they've heard it can give them breasts. Some women are afraid to eat soy protein because they're afraid it can give them breast cancer. All of these fears have to do with isoflavones, which are an estrogen-like compound that's present in soy. Let me put those fears to rest.

The isoflavones in soy foods like tofu and soy milk are weak, and in men, there is no evidence that a diet that's *moderate* in soy—the guy who drank three quarts of soy milk a day and gave himself breasts and erectile dysfunction is a bad example of moderate[21]—has any negative effects on libido, testosterone levels, or erectile function. In fact, soy has been associated with a reduced risk for prostate cancer.[22]

I've fielded questions about soy and breast cancer since I became an RD twenty years ago. The most recent research suggests that soy foods have no link to breast cancer, but rather can lower the risk of breast cancer in women.[23, 24, 25] However, *soy supplements*, which tend to be a more concentrated source of isoflavones, may not be appropriate for people who have a history of breast cancer.[26]

THE TRUTH ABOUT ORGANIC AND GMO FOODS

The choice of whether to buy organic or not is a deeply personal one.

For example, soy is the number one genetically modified crop in the world, and many people choose to avoid it because they're hesitant about consuming genetically modified foods. Most soy products are also available in organic, so if you prefer to avoid GMOs, simply choose organic soy products.

But let's be clear: There is no evidence that GMOs cause disease. Nor is there evidence that organic food lengthens life or supports health any better than conventionally produced food despite how the internet paints GMOs as evil.[27] This thinking just isn't aligned with the current science. Although some research may associate people who choose organic food with a lower risk of disease than those who choose conventional foods, this may be because organic food consumers have a more healthful diet overall.

Organic foods are significantly more expensive than conventional ones, and I take issue with websites and people who use unsubstantiated claims and fear tactics to try to convince consumers that conventional foods are toxic and poison. Biased and industry-funded activist agencies such as the Environmental Working Group (EWG) are among the worst offenders when it comes to this sort of behavior.

The truth is, organic growers use pesticides just as conventional growers do, and some of these pesticides, although "natural," are no less poisonous to humans than synthetic ones. And while recent research may have shown that children who consume organic food have lower levels of pesticides in their urine, this tiny study was flawed to the extreme.[28] First of all, it tested levels of synthetic pesticides in children's urine while they were consuming conventional food, but didn't bother to test for "organic" pesticides once the children's diet was switched to organic. The study also didn't detail what the health implications of these pesticides are, if any. The amounts in the children's urine may be far beneath the upper "safe" levels, but researchers didn't indicate any of this. The result? Readers see the headlines that scream "Conventional Foods Have Pesticides That Are Excreted in the Urine of Children!" and are immediately fearful.

Every March, the EWG puts out lists of the dirtiest and cleanest fruits and vegetable. The Dirty Dozen and Clean Fifteen lists are based on the levels of pesticides found on food during testing, which is done by an EWG-contracted lab. The Dirty Dozen is widely distributed, read, and believed, but unfortunately it's fatally flawed.

Here's why. It doesn't tell us is *which* pesticides were found, *how much* of each pesticide was detected, and what the *effects* of those pesticides are at those levels. It also doesn't tell us how the amounts found stack up against the acceptable levels of pesticides for those crops according to the EPA. I think that's pretty important information, don't you? The EWG recommends choosing organic produce over conventional, but they fail to include organic produce in the testing for the Dirty Dozen. How do we know that organics are "cleaner" than any of the foods on the Dirty Dozen list? We don't. In fact, the actual testing methodology for the Dirty Dozen and Clean Fifteen was recently exposed as lacking any sort of credibility.[29]

We can't just take information about food at face value; we need to dig deeper to see where this information is coming from and who is giving it before changing our diets. And this applies to more than just soy—it's fruits and vegetables, too.

DAIRY

As you probably saw in the earlier table, many dairy foods are a good source of protein as well as fat. They also provide us with calcium, vitamin D, and magnesium. Dairy is one of my favorite food groups because it's versatile, nutritious, and easy. Not to mention delicious. Some of the dairy products that are high in protein are Greek yogurt, ricotta, and kefir, a fermented beverage that's also good for your gut!

myth buster:

dairy causes disease.

There's a huge trend right now for going dairy-free, but in reality, most healthy people don't have to cut dairy out of their diets. Even if you're lactose-intolerant, there's always lactose-free options. Sure, if you don't tolerate dairy, it might cause you inflammation, in the same way that apples might if you didn't tolerate them. But for most people, dairy is noninflammatory and it's not an allergen or a sensitivity in the way that nutrition gurus say. After all, we've been consuming milk and milk products for centuries.[30]

Can you eat a nourishing diet without dairy? Of course! Some people have ethical concerns about dairy, which is a personal choice we don't need to address here. But for those of you who want to eat dairy and have been told to cut it out because it causes disease, I've collected the most current information so that you can make an educated—and not emotional—decision about whether to include it in your diet.

Reports of dairy foods causing phlegm, osteoporosis, cancer, and inflammation are prevalent in alternative circles, but there's absolutely no credible evidence to prove them. The China Study by T. Colin Campbell is a popular source for antidairy cancer claims, but these have been debunked. If you check the sources of many of these claims, you'll find that they're mostly biased, having come from animal welfare and activist groups. Just as they feel it's unfair to drink milk, I feel it's unfair to disseminate incorrect information and use scare tactics to try to influence people's food choices.

Others have popularized the myth that milk contains pus, in order to scare people away from consuming dairy products. The truth is that milk contains somatic cells, which are live white blood cells. Pus, on the other hand, is dead white cells, usually mixed with bacteria. If a cow has over a certain level of somatic cells in its milk, it means the animal is fighting an infection, and its milk is then not used for consumption.

I hope that puts any worries you might have had to rest. All I'll say is: If you like dairy, continue to eat it. If you don't want to eat it, you don't have to. Just don't let fear mongering and conspiracy theories make the decision for you.

ADDED PROTEINS

Adding protein to foods is more of a marketing ploy than anything else. Most foods with added protein—cereal, chips, granola bars, and cookies, for example—are still ultraprocessed and not one single bit healthier than their lower-protein counterparts. Yet shoppers snap them up because they believe in the power of protein. Even in a cookie. I'd rather you get your protein from a whole source like the ones we discussed in the sections above.

Plant milks with added protein can be a better choice than their nonprotein-fortified alternatives, simply because most plant milks are naturally so low in protein and therefore don't contribute that macronutrient to the meal or smoothie or whatever we use them in.

POWDERS

I've had clients who add protein powder to their diet on top of what they already eat in a bid to lose weight. Don't do that: Protein powders are meant to replace whole proteins and there's nothing magical about protein powder that leads to weight loss, especially when they're being added as an extra source of calories on top of your normal diet. In general, try to get your protein from whole foods because they contain other nutrients like healthy fats, vitamins, and minerals that protein powders lack.

That being said, if you use protein powders as a supplement and want to know which ones are best, here's what to look for:

- ✗ Choose a protein powder that you like. There are a lot of them that taste like shit, and people just choke them down anyhow. Don't do that.
- ✗ Find one that's low in sugar and additives.
- ✗ If you don't tolerate artificial sweeteners, watch for those on the label. Many protein powders contain them.

Plant protein powders have come a long way from their gritty, unappetizing start. Soy, rice, and hemp protein powders have been around for a while, and pea protein is the new kid on the block.

These proteins aren't complete, but as we discussed beforehand, if your diet is varied, that won't matter in the long run.

For animal-based protein powders, whey is the gold standard here. It's a complete protein that's highly digestible and absorbable. In its pure form, it tastes horrible, which is why whey protein is usually sold flavored.

Protein isolates are commonly used in plant-based protein powders, and the most common types are soy and whey. Soy-protein isolate is created by removing protein from defatted soy flakes. It's highly processed and the method used to extract protein from the soy strips away many of the beneficial nutrients, although it's high in isoflavones. It can also cause gastrointestinal, or GI, distress in some people. But as long as soy-protein isolate isn't your main source of protein, you should be fine. Whey-protein isolate is made by drying the high-protein liquid-whey by-product from dairy food production. It's high in protein but highly processed.

Soy-protein concentrate is also derived from defatted soy flakes. It's lower in protein and higher in fiber than soy-protein isolate. Whey-protein concentrate, like soy-protein concentrate, is lower in protein than whey-protein isolate. It's also less processed, and contains more fat and lactose than its isolate counterpart.

THE TRUTH ABOUT PROTEIN AND MUSCLE BUILDING

I constantly see recreational exercisers drinking protein shakes after their workouts. But do you really need a protein shake after working out? Does the extra protein build muscle? The answer is usually no.

Any sort of activity causes micro tears in our muscles. These need to be repaired and the protein we eat is what does the repairing. But slurping down a shake after an hour-long moderate workout—and by moderate I mean if you're not a competitive bodybuilder—is probably unnecessary.

There's a lot of talk about the "anabolic window," the time when the body is in muscle-building mode after a workout, and the associated protein intake that we apparently require during this time. But research shows that we have up to two hours after a workout to consume protein for optimal muscle synthesis, so if your preworkout meal was protein-rich, or your next meal is within two hours of your activity, and it contains adequate protein, you can probably do without that shake.[31,32] Instead, have a small protein-rich snack if you need something to tide you over. Contrary to common belief, you don't need to eat pounds and pounds of protein to build muscle.

There is some research suggesting that consuming protein with carbs after a workout stimulates muscle synthesis better than just protein alone. So for satiety and muscle building, consider adding a piece of fruit or another source of carb to your post-workout meal or snack!

Protein is like our body's building block. While most of us get enough of it, it's important to understand why we need it and when we should be eating it. Remember, if you eat enough protein, spaced out over the course of the day, you'll probably notice that you're less hungry and more energetic. Your meals will also be more physically satisfying.

As with everything in our diets, variety and balance are key, so don't be afraid to try incorporating plant-based proteins into your diet more often to switch things up a bit. The goal is to make meals interesting and fun, and keep you strong and healthy while you eat the foods you love.

make friends with fats

FAT. For so long, we tried to guard against it. Fat on our bodies. Fat in our food. But I want you to see fat in a different way, because fat—on our bodies and in our food—is actually a good thing.

The war against fat began in America in the 1950s, during a time when the rate of heart disease was very high.[1] Attempting to link heart disease to diet, a physiologist named Ancel Keyes began the Seven Countries Study, which seemed to prove that fat led to elevated blood cholesterol, which in turn led to heart disease and stroke. Because of this study, the American Heart Association declared in the late 1950s that a diet high in fat increased risk of heart disease. Through the following several decades, this recommendation morphed from a low-fat recommendation for high-risk people into a low-fat diet recommendation for everyone.

Fast forward to the summer of 1992. I was in university and working at a law firm in downtown Toronto. (I thought I wanted to be a lawyer, but that's a whole other story.) At lunchtime, I gave myself two options: Go into a nearby food court and order a huge fat-free frozen yogurt or go to a sandwich shop around the corner from the office and order a shrimp sandwich on plain bread with cocktail sauce. Both of those sound gross to me now, but because they were fat-free, I chose them over anything else that was available.

I also avoided foods like avocado, red meat, any dairy that wasn't fat-free, and nuts. It was the nineties, and as you know from Chapter 5 on carbs, it was a time where fat-free foods—mmm, carbs—wore an undeserved halo of health. Food companies replaced the fat in their products with sugar and starchy fillers and I, along with the rest of the population, gave myself permission to eat as much as I wanted: low-fat cookies and cupcakes and fat-free candy like licorice. All because these foods had no fat. The problem was that avoiding fat didn't make us healthier; it made us fatter and sicker. It would take years for us to realize that fat wasn't the horrible demon we thought it was.

That's not to say that the subject of fat isn't still wildly contentious. But instead of the blanket statement that "fat is bad," we now have controversy about which types of fats are best and whether all of the research on fat that has been done is actually credible. It's enough to make your head spin, which is sort of what happened when I was writing this chapter!

By the end of this chapter, you'll know what fat is, why we need it, and why the heck we can't seem to settle on a definitive answer about its links to health and disease.

WHAT IS FAT?

Let's switch gears away from our usual knee-jerk (and undeserved) negative reaction to fat and take a closer look at fat itself.

Fat as we know it is made up of different fatty acids, and is the most energy-dense macronutrient. While protein and carbohydrates each have four calories per gram, fat has nine. It's also the easiest macronutrient for the body to break down and store. Remember the Thermic Effect of Food we talked about in the last chapter? Fat's TEF is the lowest of all the macronutrients at 0 to 3 percent of calories consumed because it's so easy for our body to process fat and store it.[2] In other words, our body doesn't have to expend much energy on disassembling it and shuttling it to where it needs to go.

Our bodies are hardwired to store fat; that's how we got through times of famine in the cavewoman and caveman days. We can only store a finite amount of glycogen, which comes from carbs, and we can't store protein in its original form. The only macronutrient that we can store in infinite amounts is fat.

Now you might be thinking, "I don't want to store infinite amounts of fat," and I get it! But trust me, fat is so much more than that. It's essential to how our bodies function. The fat in the food we eat serves many different roles:

- ✗ It cushions and insulates our body so we keep warm and can sit on our butt without getting bruises!
- ✗ It slows the rate of absorption of carbohydrate when these two macronutrients are eaten together, which helps stabilize blood sugar and keep us fuller for longer.
- ✗ It transports fat-soluble vitamins A, D, E, and K. Without fat, our bodies may not absorb adequate amounts of these vitamins.

✕ It nourishes our hair and skin so they're gorgeous and all glowy-like.

✕ It makes up a large part of our brain, and is essential for cell structure and hormone production. Kind of important, right?

✕ It carries flavor in food. *Very* important. Like absolutely essential. It's impossible to be satisfied by food that doesn't taste, well . . . like anything. Like my 1992 shrimp sandwich with cocktail sauce, for example. Yuck.

✕ It makes food more satiating, meaning you feel fuller for longer.

And most important, as I mentioned above, fat is a rich source of energy, otherwise known as calories, which our bodies need to get up each day and do all the things we need to do. Fat might sound like something you want to avoid if you're trying to lose weight, but it's not, and we're going to get into that.

GUIDELINES FOR FAT INTAKE

In terms of daily requirements, it's tough for me to give you an exact number. Somewhere between 30 and 40 percent of your total calories is about right for most people, but because you're not counting calories, those percentages are relatively meaningless.

What I tell people is that they should be eating *at least* two teaspoons of fat (10 grams) at each meal for satiety and proper absorption of fat-soluble vitamins. Most of us eat more than 10 grams of fat at our meals, which is great!

Here is the fat content of some foods. This is not because I want you counting fat grams, but because I want you to be able to visualize what I mean when I talk about amounts like two teaspoons or 10 grams.

Food Amount	Fat
Slice of sprouted grain bread	2 grams
1 tsp of butter	5 grams
⅓ of an avocado	8 grams
1 tbsp of almond or peanut butter	8 grams
1 oz. cheddar cheese	9 grams
¾ cup whole-milk Greek yogurt	9 grams
Medium latte with whole milk	11 grams
Small steak	20 grams

Fat is calorie-dense, so eating a lot of it in addition to other foods may cause weight gain, but because it's so filling, most of us can replace fat-free or low-fat foods with their higher-fat counterparts and be satisfied with *less* of the full-fat versions. For example, full-fat yogurt versus a fat-free variety; a full-fat brownie versus one that's low-or-no-fat. Foods that have been engineered to be lower in fat often have more sugar or starch added to them to replicate the mouth-feel of fat. They're not healthier in any significant way. And face it: Fat-free yogurt tastes like shit. Try the full-fat stuff, enjoy it, be satisfied physically and emotionally, and move on.

When it comes to fats and health, grams of fat in what we eat isn't really the most important thing. Instead of counting fat grams, we should be focusing on our intake of healthy fats over the less healthy ones. But that's easier said than done: The science on fats and health is like a tug-of-war.

The problem with finding a definite answer about how fat—or sugar, or carbs, or basically anything out there—affects our health, is that nutrition research is usually epidemiological in nature: a study of a population and its habits over time. This is because it's unethical to keep people in a lab for years on end, controlling everything about their diet and lifestyle. But the trade-off is that population-based research is notorious for being flawed both in methodology and as a diagnostic tool because it's so tough to accurately measure cause and effect on a large group of people. What we get from most nutrition studies is more of an educated guess and a suggested link between diet and disease than a positive answer on which to base our diet recommendations.

This is precisely why nutrition science flip-flops around so much. New studies are done, but more often than not, they're flawed. For almost any nutrition topic, you can find research that argues persuasively for each side. But more often than not, we don't find any conclusions that are new and exciting. That doesn't stop the media from publishing new nutrition study reports as though they're once-in-a-lifetime breakthroughs, but that's just click-bait.

My point is, as a result of all of this noise, there's a growing mistrust of nutrition recommendations because they always seem to be changing. And the recommendations on fats are probably the worst offenders. We can't decide which fats are healthy or whether eggs give us heart attacks.[3,4] Red meat was on the "do not eat" list, now it's not.[5] So understandably, many people are still confused about which fats they should be eating or they're afraid to eat fat altogether. And this makes me very sad. We don't eat fat in isolation, and trying to micromanage what we eat can be counterproductive and frustrating.

What I know is that a healthful, complete diet contains a variety of fats, with the exception of artificial trans fats.

There are three types of fats that we eat—unsaturated, saturated, and trans fats. Unsaturated and saturated fats get their name from their molecular makeup. Without going into too much detail, saturated fats have the maximum amount of hydrogen; i.e., they are "saturated" in hydrogen. But it's important to note that every single fat out there is a combination of unsaturated and saturated fats. There are none that are 100 percent in either camp, and each fat has its own profile, meaning it has a percentage of unsaturated to saturated fats, and different amounts of each. For example, lard, one of the most notorious saturated fats, contains plenty of unsaturated fats—actually more percentage-wise than saturated ones! Olive oil, which we recommend for its unsaturated fats, has saturated fats, too. But when I talk about foods in relation to unsaturated and saturated fats, I group them by their predominant fat. For unsaturated fats, that's typically plants, and for saturated, it's typically animal fat, though there are exceptions.

There are also fats that our bodies make—cholesterol and triglycerides. We'll go through the pros and cons of all of these, but let's start with the fats we eat.

UNSATURATED FATS

MONOUNSATURATES

There are two kinds of unsaturated fats: monounsaturated and polyunsaturated. Monounsaturated fats are found primarily in plant foods, although they show up in meat for the reasons listed above. Here are examples of foods high in monounsaturated fats:

- ✗ Olives and olive oil
- ✗ Nuts and nut butters
- ✗ Seeds and seed butters
- ✗ Avocado and avocado oil
- ✗ Canola oil
- ✗ Safflower oil

These fats are commonly referred to as the good fats because much of the nutritional research associates them with health.

Monounsaturated fats appear to lower LDL cholesterol, which is considered to be a risk factor for heart disease and stroke (more on this later). While I'm not fond of categorizing foods as good or bad, I am a proponent of a diet that tips the scales in favor of unsaturated fats.

POLYUNSATURATES

Polyunsaturated fats are found primarily in vegetable oils, but also include omega-3, -6, and -9 fatty acids. Polyunsaturated fats—in particular, highly processed vegetable oils and seed oils such as canola and sunflower—have been under attack lately by low-carb dieters who believe that these fats, in any amount, cause inflammation and heart disease. My issue with these sorts of hypotheses is that most people consume vegetable oil in the form of ultra-processed and fast foods, which is a hugely confounding variable. There are other ingredients in those products that could cause the same outcome, so how can we prove that the cause is really the vegetable oils? Do we lock people in a lab and feed them nothing but seed oils for a couple of years? As I said before, we eat food, not individual nutrients. So, instead of jumping on the bandwagon and vilifying one single ingredient, consider the quality of your diet overall.

Omega-3 fats can be found in fish, which we talked about in the protein chapter. These types of omegas are DHA and EPA, otherwise known as docosahexaenoic acid and eicosapentaenoic acid. Most healthy people need 1.1–1.6 grams of omega-3s a day to support health.[6] One omega-3-fortified egg has a combined DHA and EPA amount of 0.40 grams. Here are some good sources of DHA and EPA.

Food	DHA	EPA
3 oz. cooked Atlantic salmon	1.24 grams	0.59 grams
3 oz. cooked rainbow trout	0.44 grams	0.40 grams
3 oz. light tuna (canned in water)	0.17 grams	0.02 grams
Omega-3-fortified egg	0.34 grams	

For the vegetarians and vegans out there, omega-3 fat can also be found in plant foods like flax, chia, hemp seed, and walnuts, in the form of ALA, or alpha-linoleic acid. Our bodies use only DHA and EPA, so when we consume ALA, it needs to be turned into EPA and then DHA. The process isn't efficient, though: Only up to about 15 percent of the ALA we eat is converted. If you're not eating a lot of fish or EPA/DHA-fortified foods (such as omega-3 eggs), to boost levels of absorbable omega-3 fats in your diet, you may want to consider an omega-3 supplement that's made from micro-algae, a rich source of DHA. Here are other sources of ALA.

Food	ALA
1 tbsp. flaxseed oil	7.26 grams
1 oz. chia seeds	5.06 grams
1 oz. English walnuts	2.57 grams

Omega-6 fats, which are found mostly in vegetable oils, nuts, and meats, are necessary for hair, skin, and bone health. Ultraprocessed foods also have a high amount of omega-6 fats. Because the average North American diet is full of ultraprocessed foods, it's already high in omega-6s, but it doesn't have enough omega-3s. For most North Americans, the ratio of omega-6 fats to omega-3 fats should be around 4:1, but it's currently 20:1. Having a higher ratio of omega-6 to omega-3 fats may lead to inflammation, which might be the precursor for chronic disease.[7] The research on this seems to go back and forth, but regardless, my recommendation is not to worry about getting enough omega-6s because they're so widely available in what we eat. Instead, get your fats from mostly whole foods and skip the ultraprocessed and restaurant stuff as much as possible.

Omega-9 fatty acids are actually monounsaturated—remember, all these fats are in everything to a certain extent—but unlike omega-3 and omega-6 fats, omega-9s are nonessential. This means our bodies make them, so we don't need to get them in food. Oleic acid is the most prevalent of the omega-9s, due to its presence in olive and other oils, meats, cheese, avocados, and eggs. There is some research that points to oleic acid reducing the risk of heart disease, but the link isn't conclusive.[8] Regardless, like omega-6s, you don't need to think too much about adding omega-9s to your diet.

The Mediterranean Diet is based on plants and fish, with a small amount of meat, and it appears to be one of the healthiest diets on the planet for most people.[9] This makes sense since it has mostly mono- and polyunsaturated fats, with some—but not a lot of—saturated fats.

Like I said earlier, I don't want you counting grams of fats (or grams of anything), but suffice it to say that a diet of whole and minimally processed foods, as well as food sources that are high in monounsaturated, polyunsaturated, and omega-3 fats such as fatty fish, nuts, olives, olive oil, and avocados, is what you should aim for.

SATURATED FAT

Saturated fat is commonly referred to as a bad fat and has been implicated in high cholesterol levels and risk for cardiovascular issues like heart attack and stroke since the 1960s. While saturated fat does appear to raise LDL or bad blood cholesterol, current evidence doesn't link this response to risk of heart attack, stroke, or all-cause mortality.[10, 11] A series of studies released in 2019 in the *Annals of Medicine* concluded that saturated fat has little to no effect on cardiovascular events or cancer risk. Again, these were population-based studies, which measure a trend in a population over time, not direct causation, but most current evidence seems to point in the same direction. So, contrary to what we've believed all of this time, even if saturated fat makes our blood lipid levels rise, as some studies say it does, it doesn't necessarily mean that we're bound for heart-attack city.

But this hypothesis hasn't been proved conclusively because there are just so many variables. Several studies have found that if we replace saturated fat with unsaturated fat—both monounsaturated and polyunsaturated—the risk for disease appears to be reduced.[12, 13] In other words, taking out the 17-oz. porterhouse and replacing it with some salmon. That's all well and good, but all saturated fat may not be created equal.

There are different sources of saturated fat, such as meat, dairy, and coconut oil. Each has a different saturated-fat profile and may affect our health differently. Research suggests that the saturated fat in dairy may be anti-inflammatory as opposed to the saturated fat in meat, especially processed meat.[14] Even more confounding, most nutrition studies don't separate whole meat like a steak from processed meat like bologna, even though those two foods have significant chemical and nutritional differences. That's a huge problem when looking at the quality of the evidence in that research.

Aside from all of this, saturated-fat-containing foods like meat and dairy are extremely nutritious. They contain protein, vitamins, minerals, and other valuable nutrients that can contribute positively to our health. Food isn't just about one nutrient: What it contributes to our health overall matters, too.

So, what's the verdict on saturated fat? We're just not sure. It's a fuck-tangle of contradictory research. While it seems like research doesn't prove that saturated fat causes heart disease or other major illnesses, this hypothesis hasn't been disproven either. The way each individual person reacts to saturated fat can be different, too—based on genetics, gut bacteria, activity level, and metabolism. These confounding factors muddy the waters even more.

Maybe this is why the dietary recommendations for saturated fats haven't changed in recent years. Currently, it stands at no more than 7–10 percent of our daily total calories from saturated fat. For the average person, that looks like around 14 to 20 grams. A tablespoon of butter has 7 grams of saturated fat, so according to guidelines, you'll be done after two of those.

I don't necessarily believe in these guidelines, not just because of the contradictory research, but because nobody thinks in grams; they think in food. Our overall health is the sum of the quality of the food we eat and the lifestyle we live, which is a series of trade-offs and accommodations. Some olive oil, some full-fat yogurt. Legumes, birthday cake, tons of veggies, and a glass of wine. Enjoying the food on your vacation and being more mindful when you get home. It's not all grams and weights. You need to see—and live—the whole picture.

So, let's take a step back. Saturated fat is present in many foods, but what does your diet look like as a whole? Is it made up of fast food and takeout or are you eating mostly whole or minimally processed foods? Research shows that most of the saturated fat in the North American diet comes from highly processed foods, which are typically low in fiber and plants, and high in sodium and possibly, trans fats.[15] These other ingredients may all have negative effects on our health.

Bottom line? Food is complex, and we don't eat nutrients in isolation. We should avoid picking and choosing foods based on one single ingredient, and concentrate on the totality of the food and the quality of our diet. My recommendation is to ensure that your diet has a combination of all fats, except for trans fats. While you might eat steak and butter, you should also eat foods like fish, olives, and avocado more often. Seems like a no-brainer, but people tend to eat the same foods on repeat. This isn't a healthful approach to food because, aside from overloading yourself on certain nutrients, you could be completely missing other ones that are essential for health, like certain vitamins, mineral, and fiber. And while avocado is packed with good fats, potassium, and fiber, there's something to be said for mixing things up a bit.

THE TRUTH ABOUT OILS

REFINED OILS

There are a lot of websites and nutrition gurus online who recommend staying far away from refined oils because they are toxic and harmful to our health. But is this true? Which oils are refined, anyhow? All oils are processed in some way. I mean, how would you get the oil out of olives if you didn't process them? But some oils are more processed, or refined, than others.

These include canola, soybean, corn, and vegetable oils, which are expelled from their sources using chemicals or a mill. In the refining process, they're heated, deodorized, and sometimes bleached. The high heat used during refining may decrease antioxidant and vitamin content. But does this process end up making the oils dangerous? Should you avoid canola and other refined oils?

myth buster:

heating some oils makes them dangerous.

Let's just put one thing out there right now: Heating oils enough to hydrogenate them or to make them dangerous isn't going to happen in a home kitchen while you cook your dinner. Those conditions aren't hot enough or don't last long enough to do anything harmful to fats.

Heating oils at high heat while cooking can break them down and destroy their antioxidants, particularly in extra virgin olive oil, which has the highest levels of antioxidants of any fat. In other words, while they're not dangerous, you're losing some of the nutritional benefits. Try to cook with oils that have a high smoke point and leave the low-smoke-point oils for your salads and cold dishes. Here's a list of oils and their smoke points.

Oil	Smoke Point
Extra virgin olive oil	330° F / 165° C
Butter	350° F / 176° C
Coconut oil	350° F / 176° C
Sesame oil	410° F / 210° C
Grapeseed oil	420° F / 215° C
Regular olive oil	430° F / 221° C
Peanut oil	450° F / 232° C
Sunflower oil	450° F / 232° C
Corn oil	450° F / 232° C
Canola oil	470° F / 243° C
Avocado oil	520° F / 271° C

Eh, not really. With all oils, it comes down to how much and how often you choose them. Let's put it this way: If your diet is based mostly on ultraprocessed foods, you may be consuming a large amount of refined oils (among other things). And throughout this book, we've talked about cutting back on ultraprocessed foods as much as possible, which should take care of a lot of the refined oils in your diet. If you're cooking with *only* refined oil, mix it up with other oils such as extra virgin olive oil and avocado oil. Variety is one of the hallmarks of a healthy diet.

COCONUT OIL

Coconut oil is a fat that's mostly saturated, but is made up of a lot of medium-chain triglycerides (say that three times fast, ha-ha!), or MCTs. The central thing to remember about MCTS is that they're metabolized differently than other fats; they are broken down and used as fuel faster and more efficiently, which leads some people to believe that eating coconut oil will help with weight loss. If that's you, I'm sorry: Unfortunately, studies show no significant weight-loss results from swapping coconut oil for other fats. One study did show that coconut oil increased metabolism initially as opposed to soybean oil, but after fourteen days, the effect was gone.[16]

Coconut oil isn't the health miracle that it's sometimes made out to be.[17] It has a high smoke point, so it's good for cooking, but don't go taking tablespoonfuls of it thinking it's going to make you healthier or lighter. Although it's metabolized differently, coconut oil is still as energy-dense as any other fat and will lead to weight gain if taken on top of your regular fat intake.

BUTTER

Versus margarine. Ah, the age-old debate. When it comes down to it, it's a matter of preference. I use butter because I enjoy the taste. I also don't find the research comparing the two compelling enough to make me want to switch to margarine. In fact, I don't care how many nutrition buzzwords your margarine tub has on it, there really is no evidence that margarine is significantly better for our health than butter. At least not for the amount you're probably eating.

TRANS FATS

If I was going to call any food bad—and you know I hate labels—it would be trans fats. Despite the various opinions out there on fat in general, what everyone agrees on is that trans-fatty acids can have deleterious effects on our health, including inflammation and elevated blood cholesterol levels. Currently, there's a ban on the use of trans fats in foods in both the United States and Canada.[18]

While some animals have trans fats naturally in their milk and meat, those don't seem to be as dangerous for our health as the artificial ones that are created by the food industry in a process called hydrogenation.[19, 20] Hydrogenation takes a liquid fat and turns it into a solid, which the food industry then uses to lengthen product shelf life and produce a certain taste and texture. When you see the words "hydrogenated" or "partially hydrogenated" on a food label, this means trans fats, and I encourage you to back away from the grocery store shelf.

The best example of a pure hydrogenated fat is that ubiquitous block of solid shortening that's used to make piecrust. That block wasn't always solid; it was once a liquid that was put through the hydrogenation process to create a shelf-stable solid. And while the current ban on trans fats has led companies to reformulate products like shortening, this doesn't mean these foods are trans-fat-free. There are still trans fats that hide in foods like solid shortening and some bakery products such as crackers and cookies. This is because labeling laws say that if a product has under 0.5 grams of trans fat per serving, the label can legally claim that the products contains 0 grams of trans fat and are trans-fat-free. So sneaky.

This becomes an issue if you regularly use an oil or shortening that flies under the trans-fat label radar at, say, 0.4 grams of trans fats per serving (about a tablespoon). These things add up fast, and the current recommendations for trans fats are to limit them to under 1 percent of total calories consumed. That's not a lot of wiggle room. I know I say to eat a variety of fats, but when it comes to trans fat, you should be eating as little as humanly possible. Avoid products with the words "partially hydrogenated oil" in their ingredient lists and try to limit ultraprocessed food, fast food, and store-baked goods as much as you can.

CHOLESTEROL

As promised, we're getting into cholesterol, which I've referred to throughout the chapter. Yes, cholesterol is in some of the foods we eat, but it's also a type of fat that our bodies make, and for the purposes of this chapter, that's the kind of cholesterol we want to know about. The cholesterol in our body is made by our liver, and comes in two forms: HDL, or good cholesterol, and LDL, the bad cholesterol. Most of us don't have to watch our dietary cholesterol because it's generally not a significant contributing factor in high blood cholesterol.[21]

When it comes to our LDL and HDL cholesterol levels, genetics plays a large role, and there's nothing we can do to change that. Take my friend Amber. I knew Amber when we were in our twenties, and at that time she was an avid exerciser. She ate well and led a healthy lifestyle. Amber also had very high LDL cholesterol, which is the type of cholesterol that can build up inside our arteries. So high, in fact, that her doctor wanted to put her on a cholesterol-lowering medication. But Amber didn't eat a lot of fat, she didn't smoke, and she wasn't sedentary. So what was up with her numbers? Her condition was just like so many others with high cholesterol: Her liver just made too much of it.

We can't control genetics, but because a high LDL and low HDL are still considered to be risk factors for heart disease and stroke, there are some diet and lifestyle changes we can make to optimize our cholesterol levels.

Let's start with HDL, the protective type of cholesterol. The higher the level of this cholesterol, the better, because HDL scavenges LDL and fatty acids and carries them to the liver, where they're sent out of the body. So how do we pump up our HDL levels? Fish oils, physical activity, quitting smoking, decreasing alcohol consumption, swapping refined carbs for whole grains, and limiting saturated and especially trans fats may help increase your HDL levels. Niacin, otherwise known as vitamin B3, has also been shown in some studies to increase HDL cholesterol. On the other hand, lifestyle factors such as obesity, smoking, sedentary behavior, and a diet high in alcohol, refined carbs, saturated fats, and trans fats appears to decrease HDL levels.

Not all LDL is thought to be harmful, and the difference is in particle size.[22,23] The smaller, denser LDL particles—VLDL and SD-LDL (small, dense LDL)—are far more dangerous than the light, fluffy ones, but normal blood-work tests don't generally distinguish between particle size; these results just give you a high or low LDL number overall. A lot of people who suffer heart attacks actually have LDL levels that aren't sky-high, but they have a higher number of smaller LDL particles. If you're concerned, you can ask your doctor if you need a more comprehensive test for LDL particle size. Otherwise, work on making sure your diet is optimized to re-duce LDL and increase HDL, and remember that LDL is only *one* risk factor for heart issues. There are plenty more, including your lifestyle and other health issues, such as diabetes.

Monounsaturated fats and omega-3 fatty acids appear to in-crease particle size, so a diet rich in plants can help. While plants contain fiber that helps lower cholesterol, they also contain ste-rols, which are substances that block cholesterol absorption by your body. If you're eating an otherwise healthful diet that has a lot of saturated fats, and notice that your LDL is creeping up, I'd rec-ommend that you decrease your saturated-fat intake to see if that helps.

I've provided you with a ton of detail here, but don't get too bogged down by it. The most important thing to remember is to eat a variety of fats. And fiber. Fiber. And more fiber.

TRIGLYCERIDES

You've seen me mention these throughout the book. Now we're going to dive a little deeper. Remember that I mentioned in Chap-ter 5 that triglycerides are a type of fat that floats around in your blood. They're used by our body as a source of energy. When we eat more calories at a meal than our body can use right away, the excess calories get converted into triglycerides that are then stored in our fat cells and released into the bloodstream between meals for energy. But just like anything, too much is not good, and as we mentioned before, having too many triglycerides in your blood can increase risk of heart disease. If your levels are super high, this can also precipitate pancreatitis, an inflammation of the pancreas that is brutally painful and dangerous.

Excess sugar, refined carbs, and alcohol in your diet directly contribute to the production of triglycerides. Frequent overeating does as well. If you have high triglycerides, the same recommendations apply: increase fiber; lower your sugar, refined carb, and alcohol intake; and watch your portions. Omega-3 fats may also help lower triglycerides.

Fat contributes to satiety, it carries flavor, it helps us absorb fat-soluble vitamins, and it helps our bodies produce cells and hormones. A lot of times, low-fat or fat-free foods tend to be jammed with additives and can be less satisfying than their full-fat counterparts. In those cases, I'd prefer you eat the full-fat versions.

The take-home message from this chapter is: Don't be afraid of fat. Be smart about it. We don't eat fat in isolation, so consider the quality of your diet overall instead of counting grams of unsaturated versus saturated. Chances are, if you're eating a mostly varied diet of whole or minimally processed foods, your fat intake doesn't require much scrutiny. A nourishing, healthful diet includes all fats, heavier on the mono and polyunsaturated, but including saturated ones as well.

And the last word? Fat is still the most energy-dense macronutrient out there, so avoiding it won't do you any good. For satiety, health, and satisfaction, including fat—most often the healthy types—in your meals and snacks makes a lot of sense.

8

~~rosé~~ water all day

Every single morning without fail, I head to my local coffee shop to get a huge coffee. It's my ritual, my habit, and an essential step in my day. So many of us have these rituals with what we eat and drink, but in particular with drinks, we often don't think about how they affect our nutrition overall. I mean, think about your last glass of rosé: Drinks go down so quickly, no chewing required, so it's sometimes an out-of-sight, out-of-mind situation.

Coffee, tea, smoothies, protein shakes, pop (soda for some of you), milk, juice, wine, beer, cocktails, and yes, water. The list of what we drink is long. And just like food, we've labeled certain drinks bad—like soft drinks—and others good—like green juice—but by now you know that I'm here to get to the heart of our preconceptions and misconceptions about beverages and explain exactly how what we drink impacts our nutrition. Even for those of you who don't drink pop, your cold-pressed cleansing juices and smoothies may not be living up to their hype. They also may be taking your health journey in the wrong direction.

In this chapter, I'll give you the lowdown on what fluids do in our bodies, how much we should drink, and what we should drink, and I'll bust a few myths along the way.

WHY DO WE DRINK?

We drink because we're thirsty, of course. Leave it to me to state the obvious! We drink water to rehydrate and protein shakes to refuel. We also drink for enjoyment, to relax, and to de-stress—in most of these instances I'm referring to alcohol.

But have you ever looked at the clock, noticed that it's midafternoon, and realized that you haven't had anything to drink since your morning coffee? Or worse, nothing at all? Sometimes we're so caught up in choosing the right foods, we forget about fluids. I'm guilty of this! I often catch myself thinking, "I'll just drink something in a bit," but then, three hours later, I still haven't!

Our bodies are 60 percent water, so hydration is key to making sure we're healthy, energized, and focused. Here are some bodily functions that are affected by what we drink:

- ✗ Blood pressure and heart rate. Our blood needs fluids to function properly. If you've ever been dehydrated and felt faint, it was most likely because your blood pressure was low from lack of fluid.
- ✗ Bladder health. Fluids flush out our bladder when we pee. Being hydrated can help prevent bladder infections, too.

✕ Kidney function. Fluids help produce urine, which removes waste from our blood. The kidneys also regulate our body's water balance, matching input to output.

✕ Body temperature. What we drink creates and replaces sweat. If you're not consuming enough fluids, your ability to sweat is impacted, which can lead to overheating.

✕ Joints and tissues. Fluids lubricate joints and hydrate tissues.

✕ Bowel movements. Fluids keep stool soft and easy to pass.

✕ Digestion. What we drink helps break down food. Saliva is the first step of digestion, and being hydrated helps us produce saliva. Digestive enzymes are also partly made up of the fluids we consume.

✕ Energy. Even mild dehydration can cause fatigue and sluggishness and may also affect focus.

Now here are some things water doesn't do:

✕ It doesn't burn fat. I remember an aerobics instructor in the nineties saying that we can't burn fat if we don't drink water. Turns out, she was wrong—fat burning doesn't depend on hydration, at least not directly. But being well hydrated optimizes energy levels to help athletic performance.

✕ It doesn't give us glowing, clear skin. Models and celebrities love to say this, but it's actually a myth! You'd have to be seriously dehydrated to see any effect on your skin, especially the skin on your face. Dry air can dehydrate you from the *outside*, but there's no hydrating skin from the *inside*.

As a rule, fluids clear the stomach a lot faster than solids. They're also a lot easier to consume: I can suck up a milk shake in about 5.2 seconds. Especially if they have no fat or protein in them, most

drinks go down so fast that they don't trigger our fullnes[s]
nism, leaving our bodies unaware that we've just consum[ed]
calories. As a result, we tend to drink most fluids on top of what
we eat. If you're regularly consuming sugary or caloric drinks, those
can definitely add up.

GUIDELINES FOR FLUID INTAKE

So, how much do we actually need to drink in a day? You've heard
the age-old "eight glasses of water a day" thing. Spoiler alert, it's
not based in science.[1] Although we do need fluids, as stated in the
original eight-glasses-a-day recommendation from 1945, most of
that comes from prepared foods. Many of us believe that we need
to drink eight 8-oz. glasses of fluid a day when, in fact, we can get
some of our fluids from the food we eat.

Soup, fruits, and vegetables are all rich in water. Even foods like
gelatin and ice cream hydrate us. (Did I just blow your mind?) And
unlike what I learned in nutrition school all those years ago, coffee *does* count as a hydrating fluid. YESSSS. That's great news. My
morning coffee counts for a quarter of my daily fluid intake, and
all before 9 a.m.! Perfect.

The greater news is that we don't need to count every single
drop of fluid we consume. There are ways to determine whether
you're getting enough.

So, what's your hydration status? On a break? Complicated? Try
this simple test. Pinch the top of your hand. Does the skin spring
back quickly? Or remain tented? If it's the latter, you're probably
dehydrated. Another easy test is a little more personal—checking
the color of your urine.[2] If it's dark yellow, you need to drink more;
light yellow means you're hydrated. If you're dehydrated, you might
also get a headache, have trouble concentrating, and be fatigued.[3]

If you're thirsty, that's a sign that you're on your way to becoming dehydrated, so drink up.

Our bodies lose fluid in various ways.[4,5] Urine accounts for the most losses at 1.0L–1.5L, or about three small bottles of water a day. I know, sometimes it seems like a lot more, especially during road trips. Sweating and—unbelievably—breathing account for losses between 650ml–850ml, or around 3 cups per person per day (just less than a large coffee). If you have a fever, this number gets even higher. Same if you're in a really hot environment or you're exercising strenuously. So, how much fluid we need depends on a few different things, including certain medications that may require you to drink more fluids.

For most people, I'd recommend consuming around 6 cups of fluid a day outside of your food. Let's get into the different types of fluids and their ranking from best to . . . not great.

I know you're thinking that because I'm a dietitian, I'm going to recommend you drink water and only water. That's partially correct because I do think water is the best—and cheapest—drink. But nobody drinks water all the time, because COFFEE. So let's take a look at water and your other options to see how they stack up, nutrition-wise.

WATER

I just told you that water is the best option, but what type of water? There's a ton of different kinds: tap water, filtered water, alkaline water, flavored water, and carbonated water, to name a few.

In most cities, plain old tap water is fine. There are some skeptics who believe that the fluoride in tap water is harmful to our health, but this is completely untrue—at least in the quantities that are present in our water. It's the dose that matters. Fluoride is poisonous in large amounts, but so is water, if you drink too much of it. Too much water causes hyponatremia, which is the dilution of the sodium in our blood. Electrolytes like sodium and potassium help keep our heart rate stable, so messing with that can be fatal. Most people don't reach this point, though. It's fairly tough to achieve except in exceptional cases. So while there's always someone on the internet saying that what we're eating and drinking is toxic, try not to buy into these sorts of conspiracy theories. And consider this: With tap water, unlike bottled water, you can fill and refill your own water bottle, eliminating unnecessary plastic waste.

Flavored and carbonated waters, if they're unsweetened, are also great options, especially if you're one of those people who hates the taste—or nontaste, that is—of water. Something with a little flavor or a little fizz can help you overcome that barrier.

One myth that refuses to die (and really should) is the one that says that alkaline water, which has a higher pH than normal water, is more hydrating and all-around better for us. This is complete and utter garbage, but it's a myth that the pseudoscientific acid-alkaline theory and its followers fully support.

First, alkaline water is expensive. (I smell a shifty marketing tactic.) Second, and most importantly, there isn't any evidence that it's superior to plain water.

The acid-alkaline theory dictates that what we eat can directly affect the pH of our blood and tissues, which can in turn, affect our health. The pH scale goes from 0, which is very, very acidic, to 14, which is what we call basic. The normal pH of our body is 7.4. Proponents of the acid-alkaline theory take the correct physiological process—that our body metabolizes all food into ash that's either acid or alkaline—and twist it to say that foods that break down into acid ash can cause diseases like cancer and conditions such as osteoporosis. This is untrue, and a perfect example of how perfectly legitimate science can be warped to suit an agenda.

Acid-alkaline believers try to avoid acid foods such as meat, grains, and dairy, along with some nuts and legumes. Many preach that dairy is harmful because it's an acidic food that degrades our bones, which is an assertion you may have heard but has no scientific evidence to support it. Instead, they support a diet of alkaline foods, which includes most vegetables and fruits. Fats are considered neutral.

If the acid-alkaline hypothesis were true, and we were able to control the pH of our blood and tissues with our diet, we'd die from eating pretty much anything, but thankfully, it's all a sham. No matter what we eat, the pH level of our body stays at 7.4 for healthy people because it's tightly regulated by our lungs, kidneys, and buffer system. So when we eat an acid food like dairy, meat, or nuts, our kidneys kick that extra acid out into the urine. That's all in a day's work for them, and it's all good. Our breathing and our body's bicarbonate buffer system take care of our pH, too. It's a beautifully orchestrated process, and if anything goes out of whack, you'll need a hospital, not an alkaline diet.

My issue with the acid-alkaline diet, besides the fact that it makes a complete mockery of basic physiology, is that many of the acid foods are actually nourishing. The alkaline foods are nourishing as well, but there is nothing harmful about the acid foods, especially when eaten as part of a varied diet. Eating a diet that contains acidic foods doesn't result in diseases and ill health. But many people don't know any better, and diets like these scare them into avoiding foods unnecessarily. This is not only inconvenient, but emotionally and physically unhealthy.

So now that we've covered that whole dumpster fire of a myth, let's go back to alkaline water, which is useless for anything besides hydration. If you want to spend the absurd amount of money to buy it for that purpose, be my guest, but don't fall for the claim that it's better for you.

COFFEE

Oh, coffee. I can't start my day without one. And I can't tell you how many people come to see me and admit that they drink coffee with a guilty look on their face. As if coffee is unhealthy or something! It's totally not.

We used to think that the caffeine in coffee made it a diuretic, a substance that causes increased urination, and subsequently, that drinking it was dehydrating rather than hydrating. Science has since revealed that this isn't the case, so coffee counts toward your daily fluid intake.

According to Health Canada and health authorities in the United States, the average amount of caffeine we should consume each day is under 400 mg per day.[6] (Slice that number in half if you're pregnant or nursing.) While the amount of caffeine in coffee is determined by the bean roasting process—light roast coffees are higher in caffeine—the average 8-oz. cup of coffee contains around 95 mg of caffeine.[7]

Caffeine, in appropriate doses, can help you concentrate and enhance athletic performance. I used to take caffeinated gels during marathons, and I'd never run a race without having a cup of coffee first. Coffee also has antioxidants that may contribute to our health.[8]

Of course, consuming too much caffeine can cause jitteriness, headaches, insomnia, and anxiety, and if you have cardiovascular issues, you should watch your intake.[9] We're all different in terms of our tolerance of caffeine, and the more caffeine you consume, the higher your tolerance gets. If you find yourself feeling like crap or like you need to be peeled off the ceiling after that second cup of coffee, try tea . . . or water.

It's not only about the caffeine, it's about what you put into your coffee. I'm not going to say that you should be drinking your coffee black, but if you're a fan of syrupy, creamy coffee drinks, it's best to limit them and treat them like a dessert. That said, I've been known to recommend lattes to clients for snacks! A medium latte contains 16 grams of protein, 190 calories, 150 mg of caffeine, and 7 grams of fat. The protein and fat in the drink will help with satiety, and the milk is a source of calcium.

myth buster:

caffeine burns fat.

There are a ton of caffeine products on the market that promise to burn fat by increasing your metabolism. The sources of caffeine in these products vary—some contain straight caffeine while others are from "natural" sources like green coffee bean, yerba maté, guarana, and camellia.

But this claim isn't supported by research. While caffeine can cause our metabolic rate to rise, this is only temporary, and the resulting calorie burn isn't significant enough to cause weight loss. The same goes for other "fat-burning foods" such as chili peppers and freezing-cold water. These have a short, transient effect on our metabolism, but no appreciable weight loss results. No foods burn fat.

TEA

Tea is a good alternative to water for hydration. And herbal teas, such as peppermint and hibiscus, and black teas are a low- or no-caffeine alternative to coffee, if that's what you're looking for.

Tea is sort of having a moment right now, but be careful about some of the health claims. The wellness industry has co-opted it as the latest cure-all, and the promises are a little over-the-top. Some of the usual tea suspects and their "benefits" are:

- Green tea and fat burning
- Teatoxes and weight loss
- Mushroom tea and stress reduction
- Black tea and antioxidants

The thing to remember about these teas is that the dosage of whatever active ingredient you're getting may not be sufficient to yield any benefits. The active ingredients also haven't been studied that much. Adaptogens like holy basil, reishi, and even turmeric are really popular, but the claims made about their effect on immunity, stress adaptation, and overall health are far ahead of the actual science.

I have to make a special shout-out to detox teas, otherwise known as teatoxes. Most of these are herbal diuretics and laxatives that hide behind "natural" ingredients. Trust me when I tell you that natural and herbal laxatives will give you the same cramping and diarrhea as their nonnatural counterparts. These products can cause serious dehydration, heart arrhythmias, and other side effects. Plus, any weight you lose from them will be water and poo, which of course will come back as soon as you eat or drink anything. Most importantly, if you pee and poo, and have a liver and two kidneys, there's no reason to detox anything. It's all taken care of by your body. Isn't nature wonderful? Save your money.

myth buster:

drinking fluid with meals dilutes stomach acid and impairs digestion.

I guarantee you've heard this one before. The pH of our gastric environment is usually around 3, which is highly acidic. This is completely normal. If our stomach wasn't acidic, we wouldn't be able to break food down properly. And that's exactly what the people who buy into this myth believe: that fluids should only be consumed before or after meals to avoid weakening stomach acid.

This myth flies in the face of basic physiology. The acidity of our stomach contents is controlled by parietal cells, which are special cells in our gut that maintain a healthy pH balance. When they sense the pH of the stomach is becoming less acidic (which isn't great for digestion), they secrete hydrochloric acid to balance things out. So, drink as much as you want while you eat, and don't listen to people who spout this sort of nonsense.

Also: if this myth was true, how would we digest soup?

SMOOTHIES AND PROTEIN SHAKES

As a rule, I don't advise people to include smoothies or smoothie bowls—which are essentially spoonable smoothies with toppings—in their diet on a regular basis, especially if they're the store-bought ones. Often made with frozen yogurt or a ton of fruit, these tend to be sugar bombs with a health halo. I hate to break it to you, but an acai bowl isn't healthy. It's like a one-pound bag of frozen fruit, pureed and served with pretty toppings. Yes, acai has fiber and antioxidants in it, which are good for you, but that doesn't mean we should eat 3 cups of it topped with granola, peanut butter, and coconut, which is usually what happens because acai is low in sugar and generally tastes, well, like dirt. So stores blend it with other stuff like juice and sweeter fruit—a sugar explosion.

Even homemade smoothies can be devoid of protein and over-the-top with sugar and calories. A lot of people love their break-fast smoothies, but say they're hungry two hours later. The most common reason is that the smoothies they're making don't have enough protein to keep them full. You might make a smoothie that contains almond milk, which has almost no protein, and a mix-ture of fruits, which are entirely carbs, and some peanut butter for protein. Another popular one is almond milk with fruit, spinach, and a couple tablespoons of hemp seeds or nuts. Even though these drinks do contain protein from the nuts, hemp hearts, or peanut butter, it's nowhere near the 20–25 grams of protein I recommend at meals. To get there, you'd have to include around five to six table-spoons of peanut butter, six tablespoons of hemp hearts, or ¾ cup of almonds.[10, 11, 12] Yikes. Each one of those things would send the calories through the roof . . . and can you imagine eating all that peanut butter? You'd have to jackhammer the smoothie off the roof of your mouth. Whole foods like nuts and seeds are packed with nutrition, but it is possible to eat too much of them.

One way to get more protein is to swap out the almond milk for Greek yogurt, but if you still find your smoothies don't keep you full for long enough, then the smoothie, even with the protein it contains from the yogurt, may be leaving your stomach too quickly to keep you satiated. In other words, your body isn't registering that you're eating food because, well, technically, you're not. Blending your food into a drink pulverizes the fibers that you'd otherwise be chewing, which contributes to the satiety of your meal. Although a smoothie will have more fiber than a juice, it's still less than whole foods. It's just a function of drinking, not chewing, your food. So, consider having the smoothie for a snack and eating something solid for breakfast instead.

If you love smoothies and smoothie bowls, there is a healthier way. For smoothies, try starting with a scoop of low-sugar protein powder, Greek yogurt, cow's milk, or silken tofu for protein, then adding some greens and a small portion of fruit (no more than ¾ cup). Cacao nibs or a couple of tablespoons of nuts give a crunchy texture. For a healthier acai or smoothie bowl, try making your own by using Greek yogurt, an acai packet, some greens such as spinach, kale, or arugula, and lower-sugar toppings like plain coconut or nuts in a small bowl. Small being the operative word here: The acai and other smoothie bowls on Instagram are humongous and aren't really a good representative of what constitutes a nourishing meal with a reasonable amount of sugar and protein. In fact, I'm pretty skeptical about whether the influencers who post them are actually eating them (and I've seen in real life that many of them don't).

GREEN JUICE

Celery juice. That kale liquid that looks like sewage water. "Detox" greens. Most people drink these for the purported health benefits and cleansing properties. I'm sorry to tell you that despite what the companies selling them say, these green juices don't detox or cleanse or reset your body, restore your metabolism, clean the fat from your life, and all the other ridiculous claims I've seen being made about these sorts of regimens. It's all malarkey. And it goes back to the lie of diet culture that some foods are clean and some foods are dirty, that we aren't good enough the way we are, and that there's something wrong with our body, which can be solved if we submit to some sort of punishing detox.

Yes, green juices do contain water and vitamins, but drinking a glass of twelve-dollar sewage-water kale cleanse is not equivalent to eating solid vegetables. Drinking juice instead of eating food isn't healthier because juicing produce takes the fiber out of the end product and delivers a drink that's mostly water (and sugar, if you're juicing fruits). I know what you're thinking: "But, Abby, you want me to drink water!" I do, but it's better to chew these foods so you feel satiated—you'll still get the water and all the vitamins.

On top of that, green juices are super expensive, whether you're buying them premade or buying the raw ingredients and doing it yourself. You're better off saving your money and drinking water.

DIET AND SUGAR-FREE DRINKS

What happens when you take the sugar out of your fav drinks? Does it make them a great alternative to their sugary cousins? Well, yes and no.

Sweet foods and drinks—whether sugar-sweetened or artificially sweetened—when consumed throughout the day, blunt our taste for sweets. In other words, we get used to having everything sweetened, and then we expect it. Also, some sweeteners are several times sweeter than sugar, so we build up a tolerance to sweet things, especially ones that are less sweet, which can lead to wanting to sweeten everything we eat. If you feel as though you need to sweeten a lot of your food, or can't drink something unless it's sweet, teach your body to expect less sweet by cutting down the sweet you eat, slowly and consistently. For example, if you typically have two sugars in your coffee, try having just one. And if you're drinking more than one diet soda or artificially sweetened drink a day, I'd recommend trying to cut down as much as you can.

Now, about those sweeteners. I hear a lot of shitty science being thrown around by people who believe that diet drinks are toxic garbage. Our consumption of artificial sweeteners *has* increased exponentially in the past few decades, but there is no evidence that sweeteners are making us fatter and sicker, which is what a lot of people on social media want you to believe.

Most studies on artificial sweeteners either have been done on animals or are population-based, giving us little usable information to prove that they're unsafe. Sucralose has been linked to migraines, but as far as the connection between sweeteners and cancer, gut health, inflammation, obesity, diabetes, and anything else relevant to health, there is no solid evidence.

While eating a lot of artificial sweeteners increases our tolerance to sweet things, you're not going to keel over from the occasional diet soda. So, choose whichever sweetener you prefer, but just use as little as possible. That way, you'll get used to tasting whatever it is you're eating or drinking, all the while weaning yourself off of overly sweet foods and drinks.

FRUIT JUICES

From the glass of freshly squeezed orange juice at breakfast to the cold-pressed exotic elixir at your gym juice bar, I feel the same way about fruit juice as I do about green juice: I'd rather you eat the whole fruit.

Fruit juices, even those without added sugar, are a concentrated source of natural sugar without any of the fiber from the fruit. Like green juices, fruit juices do contain some vitamins and they are hydrating. But for the calories they contain, I'd really rather you limit your consumption of them and chew your fruit instead.

Try choosing them less often or cut down by mixing the juice with carbonated water or tap water. The same goes for serving juice to kids—limit to ½ cup a day and cut it with water. Don't let them suck on a juice-filled bottle every day as this can damage their teeth.

SUGAR-SWEETENED BEVERAGES

Grande iced mocha. Kombucha. Lemonade. Some of you love a can of Coke when you're eating pizza or a pumpkin-spice latte when fall weather hits. And this isn't a big deal. It goes back to one of the reasons we eat and drink: enjoyment.

The thing to keep in mind is that these beverages are generally loaded with sugar and not much else. Sure, a PSL has milk in it, but it's also super sweet, and whether you're trying to lose weight or simply want to eat a more healthful diet, the regular consumption of sugary drinks isn't a great idea, so try to not make it a habit.

ALCOHOL

For many of us, alcohol is a part of our regular diet, whether it's a glass of red wine with a nice steak dinner, a beer or two with chips as we watch sports, or a champagne toast to celebrate a special occasion. I'm not here to tell you that you can't have that cocktail with your colleagues after work, but if you're trying to lose weight or just improve your health, it's important to look at your alcohol consumption.

The CDC's guidelines for alcohol consumption are:[13]

✖ No more than 1 drink a day for women.

✖ No more than 2 drinks a day for men.

The Canadian recommendations are a little more generous:[14]

✖ 7–10 drinks a week for women, with no more than 2 drinks on most days.

✖ 14–15 drinks a week for men, with no more than 3 drinks on most days.

And finally, a drink is equivalent to:

✖ 12 oz. of beer

✖ 5 oz. of wine (That's a pretty small glass, FYI.)

✖ 1.5 oz. of liquor (Your margarita probably has two drink equivalents in it.)

For reasons we'll get into now, I think these guidelines are rather lenient. Here's why.

Alcohol really has no nutritional value to speak of—it's sort of tied with sugar-sweetened beverages in that regard. Sure, red wine has resveratrol, an antioxidant that purportedly extends life. But studies on that are small, short, and mostly based on actual resveratrol supplements, not on wine.[15] Even if it was the case, you can get the same antioxidant from eating grapes, blueberries, pistachios, and peanuts, and those foods are far more nourishing and come with a lot less physical risk.

Not only does alcohol contain calories that are completely non-nutritive, it can make us eat more, too.[16] Remember leptin, the hormone that curbs our appetite? Alcohol may inhibit its effects, and the effect of another hormone called GLP-1, causing us to feel hungry. It also lowers blood sugar, which again, makes us crave food—especially carbs. That's why once you get home after a long night of partying, you're probably going to snack on everything in sight. Or you'll be snacking the entire next day. Been there, done that.

Think about it this way: Let's say you drink an average of about eight drinks a week, which a lot of my clients do. Let's say that these drinks are rather hefty pours of wine, also very common. This habit will contribute around 1,200 calories to your diet weekly. Remember, these are highly absorbable calories that don't register as food and may cause you to eat more. In a month, those calories add up to just under 5,000. That's the equivalent to a hell of a lot of solid, nourishing food, food that won't make you feel like shit in the morning.

If you're not concerned about losing weight, consider the effect of alcohol on your overall health. Because it's a diuretic, alcohol dehydrates us, raising our heart rate, dropping our blood pressure, and making us fatigued, headachy, and dizzy. Alcohol is also an ir-ritant that aggravates the stomach lining, making us feel nauseous, and it affects sleep, so we don't drop into the REM stage, causing grogginess and problems with concentration.

Alcohol affects women differently than it does men.[17] We get drunk faster and our livers are more susceptible to damage. A 2015 study in the *BMJ* showed that moderate alcohol consumption— more than one drink per day—may also increase risk for breast cancer.[18] And according to the Canadian Institute for Health Infor-mation, the rate of women who died from causes linked directly to alcohol—such as liver disease—has increased by 26 percent since 2001.

I don't want to shame you for drinking, but rather present the research that's out there so you can rethink the amount of alcohol you drink and consider how you might cut down on your intake. Sure, a glass or two of wine when you have dinner with friends is A-OK, but half a bottle of wine a night is overkill.

In general, alcohol is becoming a more accepted part of our culture—a reward after a hard day of work or parenting—and it's sold with the subversive message that it will smooth the edges, give you a sense of belonging, and can be a part of a healthy life. There are even beer yoga classes, beer runs, and bars at some gyms. "Mommy's juice" and other tongue-in-cheek phrases are common decorations for aprons, wineglasses, and memes. As with food, I want you to be aware of the effects of alcohol advertising and the reasons why you're consuming the drinks you are.

If you drink socially and occasionally for enjoyment, that's okay, but it's different if you feel compelled to out of habit or custom. While we all have our vices, if you find yourself reaching for alcohol on a regular basis, I'd encourage you to be conscious of what purpose it's serving you. Like we talked about earlier, it's normal to have emotional-eating triggers and alcohol is something that's often consumed out of emotion, especially to relieve stress. If you're uncomfortable with the amount of alcohol you're consuming, I'd encourage you to dig deeper into what's behind your drinking as you did with the hunger and fullness scale.

Phew! Never in a million years did you think I'd have so much to say about fluids, right? Often they're just something we take in, not what we think about . . . at least not as much as we think about food.

But when it comes to losing weight and being healthy, often making small modifications to what we drink can have a huge impact. In fact, it's the number one change I ask my clients to make and it's usually the easiest because many of us drink caloric beverages like pop, wine, and PSLs for enjoyment, not to fill our stomachs. For someone who drinks five cans of Coke a day, limiting their intake to one isn't really the end of the world, but the impact it makes on their weight is, in most cases, huge.

And remember, no drink is off-limits, but hydration is the goal, and in most cases, water is the best candidate for the job. You don't have to chug 64 oz. of it either. Coffee counts. So does ice cream.

high-value eating

We've been on a journey, haven't we? Now that we've learned how to repair our relationship with food and covered the basic building blocks of food and drinks, it's time to introduce you to high-value eating. This is the chapter that's going to answer all of those "But what do I eat?" questions that you keep asking in your head. Yes, we've come to that part of the book. Let's do this!

WHAT IS HIGH-VALUE EATING?

I went through a few renditions of what I wanted my eating method to be called. I didn't want anything diet-related—obviously—so out went anything with the word "diet" or "plan." I wanted a name that reflected my true philosophy that *food and eating should add to your life, not take away from it, in every way: emotionally, physically, socially, and financially.*

"High value" speaks to my cost-benefit way of approaching food and life in general: that a life spent dieting costs us more in all those ways I listed above than it's worth. It also describes the value in knowledge gained because I'm teaching you to make your own decisions about food instead of giving you meal plans and telling you what to eat and what not to eat. That means this is doable. It's customizable. It works *for* you, not the other way around.

High-value eating means eating a diet of food that nourishes, not only physically, but emotionally. It satisfies you and makes you happy, and has zero tolerance for guilt and shame. Instead, high-value eating honors our most primal instincts: to feed ourselves, to gather around food, and to find pleasure in flavor and taste. A high-value meal is satisfying, and it often contains protein, healthy fats, fiber, and plants. Not always, though: Some high-value meals contain Oreo cookies and pizza.

That's because high-value eating doesn't operate from a place of restriction; instead, it adds foods to your diet and recognizes that some foods may not be the most physically nourishing, but still bring us joy. I truly believe that we don't have to stop eating any certain type of food in order to be healthy. When we restrict, we just fall hard eventually. So these foods can be consumed responsibly, but are not excluded from our routines. No food is excluded.

High-value eating doesn't count calories or macros, or assign labels to food like "clean" and "good." It spits in the face of diet culture and rejects all of its principles. So there!

Most of the people I've counseled aren't great with the loose permissiveness of "eat when you're hungry, stop when you're full," and I don't blame them because I'm the exact same way. Although guidelines like those can be valuable, they leave a lot of room for interpretation. The hunger scale, which we discussed earlier, is a valuable tool that should be used in conjunction with high-value eating, but it doesn't answer the question "What should I eat?" There's no one-size-fits-all response to that. It's different for everyone, which is why I'm not giving you meal plans and those dreaded lists of do and don't foods that other books contain. Those don't exist in my world, and they shouldn't exist in yours either. I'm also not going to give you a grocery list because although I always see them in nutrition books, I feel like they're an insult to your intelligence. You don't need a list of which vegetables to buy.

Let's start with my Ten Tenets of High-Value Eating.

1. Be a pencil, not an eraser.

I live and die by this theory because over the past twenty years or so, I've seen (and lived) far too many eating plans and diets that take things away from us unnecessarily. It has become so ingrained in our culture that when I go to a party or some other event and people hear I'm a dietitian, they always want me to tell them what *not* to eat. "What do I need to cut out of my diet?" they ask me. It's literally never "What can I add back?" I think it's pretty sad that we're coming at food and eating from this perspective. But that's diet culture for you, always saying no to the foods you love, and then giving you lame reasons why.

People, in general, respond far better to making changes when they are positive ones, which is why I always start by telling clients what to add back into their diets. I love seeing the look on their faces when I do this. It's like a combination of disbelief and utter joy when they hear that they can actually eat yogurt and bread and whatever else they had cut out because someone unqualified told them to. You can't heal your relationship with food if you're focusing on what you CAN'T eat, foods to "detox" from, and foods that are "harmful," etc.

Being a pencil means adding food back into your diet; in doing that, you will fix your relationship with food, your body, and your eating. Food goes from being a loaded, stressful thing to something peaceful and fun. Adding food back in this way reaffirms that eating can be enjoyable, pleasurable, and nonpunitive.

Right now, I want you to think about all of the foods you're not eating. That you've been told not to eat, that you think are fattening, toxic, or bad. Someone may have told you that eliminating these foods can help you lose weight or that eating them can cause weight gain. (If you have a medical condition and your doctor or allergist MD has recommended cutting out certain foods, that's okay. Listen to them. This is a different story.)

Let's take a step back and put all of those rules and thoughts of forbidden foods into a little box. We're going to forget about them because they're not based on truths. They're made up by people who use pseudoscience to sell us a product or a diet. Rules like these take away from our lives and they don't make us any healthier. They just make us feel like we're being punished. That's a really shitty way to live your life, don't you agree?

"But, Abby!" you say. "If I add back bread/nightshades/Oreos/dairy/my mom's Thanksgiving stuffing, I'm going to gain weight!"

This is what some of you are thinking, and I know it because I've been doing this for a very long time. And my answer? If you add foods back and don't make anything off-limits, you won't feel like you have to overeat them. If you eat normally and from a high-value perspective, your body weight will naturally fall where it's supposed to.

Remember, we all have that comfortable weight that our body likes to be at. Maybe you think yours is too high. Maybe you don't.

I'm not saying you can't fight genetics, environmental factors, and all the other things that determine body weight. I'm saying that if you're haggling with your body over a few pounds, it's probably not worth it.

Adding foods back into your diet and accepting your natural weight might involve a bit of a trade-off, but I promise that the benefits are worth it. Ask yourself these questions:

✗ What if you added all of these foods back and you gained some weight?

✗ Would you be willing to trade a few pounds for never having to restrict food again?

✗ Would you be willing to accept your body at its natural, comfortable weight if it meant that you didn't have to play tug-of-war with it anymore?

✗ Or, would you be content to fight your body over a few pounds for the foreseeable future?

If you have a lot of weight to lose, adding foods back into your diet and not dieting can also normalize your weight. You, too, might be fighting to sustain unrealistically low calorie levels and food restrictions. These are battles that nobody wins. At least, not for the long term.

So, lay down your weapons, people. We need to call a truce. We're still making changes here: The types of foods you're eating and your meal scheduling might change, but the volume of food you're eating will probably stay the same.

Right now, let's do this pencil thing. If you are a chronic dieter, add back everything to your diet that you unnecessarily cut out because diet culture told you to. The usual suspects are wheat, gluten, and dairy, but there are so many more. Keto dieters who are done with being on that plan can add back grains and fruits. Those of you who have been slogging along on Paleo and Whole30 can add back dairy and legumes. And if you haven't been on any specific diet in particular, don't restrict yourself from any type of food.

2. Eat whole or minimally processed foods when you can.

Many people refer to foods as whole or processed, but I prefer the terms "whole," "minimally processed," and "ultraprocessed," which are used by the NOVA food classification system. NOVA was developed in consultation and testing with scientists in numerous countries, and unlike the nebulous influencer definitions that exist on social media, NOVA definitions are specific and evidence-based:

- ✖ Whole foods are those that are in their original, natural form. Whole fruits and vegetables, fresh or frozen, are in this category. Frozen foods are technically processed, but if they're simply whole foods that are frozen, then I call them whole.
- ✖ Minimally processed foods have been altered lightly, such as hummus, yogurt, milk, or canned tuna.
- ✖ Ultraprocessed foods have been completely altered from their original ingredients in processes such as refining and have many additives, such as deli meat, most crackers, and microwave meals.

High-value eating is based on making your diet full of whole and minimally processed foods, then throwing some ultraprocessed foods in there. Roughly 75 percent of the food you eat should be whole or minimally processed. If you can't manage that, try it with roughly 50 percent of your food. Because sometimes "good enough" is the best option!

There's another reason why I use these three terms. You've probably heard plenty in the media about the goodness of whole, unprocessed foods and the badness of processed foods, but it's important to clear up a few things.

First, the privilege that's attached to these terms. I want to ensure that high-value eating is accessible to everyone, which is why I don't recommend niche and expensive foods. Hey, if you want to eat French butter, go right ahead. But the stuff from your regular supermarket is good, too. And it's also why I don't recommend making ultraprocessed foods off-limits. I think we all understand that eating foods that are closest to their natural forms is ideal, but doing this for every food at every meal isn't realistic.

There are a lot of influencers on social media who talk about how their diets contain only "real food." I can't stand that. It's elitist and gross. It puts a morality-based judgment on food that I completely don't agree with. In my world, "real food" is anything that's edible. The opposite of "real" is "fake," and I refuse to classify any food under that term. If someone can't afford what some people call a "real food diet," they're no less of a person. Their diet isn't toxic or bad.

Second, when people condemn processed foods, they fail to acknowledge that most foods we eat are processed. Milk is processed when it's pasteurized. Almonds are processed when they're shelled. Peanut butter is processed peanuts. Just because something is processed doesn't mean you shouldn't eat it.

And yet this idea abounds on the internet with myths such as "don't eat food that has a bar code" or "don't buy foods with any more than five ingredients." Who buys only foods without bar codes? Even my apples have bar codes on them! The number of ingredients in a food product does not reveal if the food is a nourishing choice. Sure, many ultraprocessed foods have a lot of ingredients, but so does my mom's legendary brisket. These unfounded, privileged suggestions might be great for someone who grows and makes all their own food, but that's not me, and I'm pretty sure that's none of you either.

3. Understand your lifestyle.

Are you a breakfast eater? Do you work long hours? Do you travel a lot, or have a long commute? If you can anticipate barriers before they occur, they'll be a lot easier to get around as we discussed in Chapter 4.

So what does this look like from a high-value eating perspective? For example, if you know that you have a long commute, you might include a high-protein snack before leaving the office in the evening. Or, if you travel a lot for work, you might incorporate frozen vegetables more than fresh ones, so your greens are always available and ready when you are.

Small changes add up to huge ones, so remember that whatever you do doesn't have to be a complete overhaul all at once to what you eat. Keep in manageable.

4. Make peace with your preferences.

Eat what you love, not what you think you should eat. If you hate broccoli, don't eat it because you think you need to—there are hundreds of other options. No one or two foods are going to make or break your diet.

Remember your list of nonnegotiables? Have a look at that now with everything you've learned in mind. You'll want to tweak your diet to accommodate them. For example, if your nonnegotiable is having two sugars in your coffee every morning, which sugary foods are you willing to decrease your intake of to make room for the coffee sugars?

5. Replace the replaceable.

Most of us glide through the grocery store, picking up the same things each week out of habit. Take the time to really think about what nourishes you physically and emotionally. Which foods are serving you and which foods aren't?

If you usually buy a lot of ultraprocessed or sugary items, try leaving out the ones you don't absolutely love. You can always get them if you really want them; they're not going away, I promise. And don't buy these foods "for your kids or your spouse" because "they like them" if you know deep down that you're probably going to be the one eating them. If your kids love cookies, buy a kind that you don't love and leave it at that. If you know that your husband or wife loves ice cream and Lucky Charms, but you can't lay off them, don't bring them into the house.

It's not just your food habits that should be changing; the entire household's habits should be tweaked, too. Remember that this is about your health *and* the health of your family. That's not to say that ultraprocessed foods need to be cut out entirely, but balancing them with more nourishing foods is what we're aiming for. So buy what you love, and leave the other things behind.

6. Be intentional and quiet that "diet" voice.

Maybe you want some fries with your lunch. Or, your mom's brownies. Or, that gelato that looks so good on a summer night. Eat with intention. Be aware of how you feel, what you crave, and what you eat.

Don't tell yourself that you're not going to eat something because it's bad, then go back and forth about it until you break down and eat it anyway. THERE ARE NO BAD FOODS. Food is food. We don't eat numbers, so choose food for its beauty, taste, and quality. Eating should be a peaceful experience. While there are foods that you might want to eat less often, they aren't bad and choosing those foods doesn't make you a bad person. Even when you choose these foods for breakfast sometimes. Even when you feel like you've overdone it with those types of foods that week. This makes you normal. This is normal eating.

Remember what normal eating is?

- Eating in a consistent and sustainable way.
- Feeling hunger when we start eating and feeling satisfied when we stop.
- Understanding that sometimes we overeat, and when it happens occasionally, that's okay.
- Choosing foods that most often support our long-term physical and emotional health.
- Eating a wide variety of foods.
- Feeling peace, not guilt and shame, around food.
- Knowing that on some days we'll need more food, and on others, less.

Guilt and shame make us feel like shit, and they're completely counterproductive. Eat your food, enjoy it, taste it, and then move on. No punishment, no feeling bad. Because . . .

7. It's about balance.

Balance is key. But don't think that this balance can be achieved every day of your life, because that's unrealistic. Some days are more nourishing than others. Protein, fiber, and vegetables rule, but some days, so does cake. Food should be both physically and emotionally satisfying, which is why choosing foods you enjoy is important.

Balance may be different for everyone, but it looks sort of like this:

✂ If you have dessert after lunch, try not to have it after dinner.

✂ If you don't have any greens at lunch, pile them on at dinner.

✂ If you've been on vacation for a week and had about zero grams of fiber the entire time, go back to your normal eating habits once you return home.

✂ If you really want a stack of pancakes for breakfast, eat a protein-rich lunch and supper.

No joke, it will all fall into place. Punishing yourself with undereating, overexercising, or negative self-talk when you eat less nourishing foods is a recipe for disaster. Forget that and just gently go back to eating a diet of mostly whole and minimally processed foods.

8. Be flexible.

Honestly, I think this is one of the most important tenets of all: flexibility.

A lot of diets ask you to be rigid in your food choices and thinking: No grains. No bad foods. You must have certain foods at certain times on certain days. That shit doesn't work for anyone, at least not in the long term. All it does is make you perpetually anxious and on guard, unable to relax about situations where you might inadvertently cheat on your diet. And that doesn't feel good at all. Like, ever.

Flexibility goes hand in hand with balance in that sometimes you're going to be in a place where there's no vegetables. Or, you may have wanted eggs for breakfast but the only thing in your fridge is pasta. You might be out with your friends, who want to split a huge pizza when you planned on having salad. Whatever, you know what I'm saying. Flexibility is a mind-set that understands and trusts your body.

9. Eat for you, not for everyone else.

Keep your eyes on the prize here: changing your eating habits for you. Which means, pull yourself back when you see diet trends pop up that you'd normally jump on. Even if everyone in your office, group of friends, and Facebook seems to be into them, you need to do what's good for YOU. This means being consistent and letting go of the compulsion to compare your diet to everyone else's, and to hop on and off the fad train, which only holds you back and makes you feel shitty. Trendy doesn't necessarily fit into your goals or your wallet.

10. Eat according to your hunger, not the clock.

A lot of books about nutrition and eating will have you eating three meals and three snacks a day. Not this one. That's not to say that the three and three won't work for you, but I want to open your mind to the fact that we sometimes eat because we think we're supposed to.

For example, I've had many clients who use their afternoon break as a run to a coffee shop for a latte or a muffin, even though they're not really hungry at the time. "But it's a good excuse to get up from my desk!" they tell me.

"But you're not hungry! Can you not just take a walk instead?" I say to them.

The same thing goes for meals. Somehow, when the clock

strikes noon, it's automatically lunchtime, whether we're hungry or not. But why? Sometimes—especially in some workplaces—lunch is a social thing. You don't want to sit there working while your colleagues are in the lunchroom or at a restaurant, taking well-needed break time. But being aware of your hunger level and eating accordingly—either delaying or eating less if you're not that hungry—is smart. Remember the tenet of being intentional? It applies here, too. Eating meals and snacks out of habit, even when you're not that hungry, doesn't make much sense.

One of the best examples of this tenet is breakfast. When I first started as an RD, I used to tell people to always eat breakfast. It felt weird, though, to tell people to eat when so many of them weren't hungry in the morning. I've since changed my tune.

First off, start with the principle of eating when you're hungry. If this means that you take a pass on breakfast because you just don't get hungry until 11 a.m., then that's fine. Research about the benefits of breakfast isn't conclusive, and it's best not to force yourself to eat, especially if you're trying to tune in to your body's natural cues. "Breakfast is the most important meal of the day" is a saying that was invented in the 1900s by John Harvey Kellogg to convince people that his newly developed cereal was an essential start to their day. It's not exactly science-based. More like a marketing ploy. So let's not fall for it.

I have nothing against breakfast. If you're a breakfast eater, keep eating it! If you're not, just make sure that you listen to your body and eat when you feel hungry. The issues with skipping meals—either breakfast or others—can be hunger later on in the day or inadequate nutrient intake (especially if you skip frequently). While intermittent fasting is popular now, don't automatically skip breakfast because you think it's going to help you lose weight. Some people can skip a meal such as breakfast without overcompensating later on in the day; others become ravenous when their body starts looking for the nutrition it missed in the morning.

If you skip breakfast and overcompensate later in the day, then you might want to try adding in breakfast to see if that helps. Think about it this way: You might be better eating something in the morning rather than overeating later at night to make up for skipping breakfast.

If you eat breakfast but still find yourself snacking continuously at night, bring out that hunger journal. Think about why you're eating. Remember there is true hunger and emotional hunger. Are you hungry or are you trying to fill another need? Look at the hunger and fullness scale. Where does your hunger sit on it? If you're not truly hungry—i.e., around a 4–5 on the scale, what do you need right now?

When you reach for food, try to be aware of how you're feeling. You don't have to be starving hungry to eat, but if you tend to overeat or eat mindlessly, being conscious of why you're eating is always a good exercise. It's true that normal eating sometimes means that you'll eat for emotion, pleasure, or experience instead of true hunger, but knowing how often you do this can help you determine whether you need other coping mechanisms or ways to connect with people.

Try to get used to using your body's cues to time meals and snacks, rather than the clock. If your day is built around meal and break times and you don't have much control over that, try to adjust your intake according to how you feel at the time.

A GUIDE TO HIGH-VALUE EATING

High-value eating is not only about having a good emotional relationship with food and eating, but also choosing foods that are physically nourishing and satisfying. It's important to ensure that your meal has the right balance of macronutrients to be physically satisfying. Here's what that looks like.

MEALS

1. Prioritize protein.

Each meal you eat should revolve around a protein source for satiety. You'll want to choose your protein, then build your meal out from there. Plant or animal, you want a high-quality source, whether that's chicken or chickpeas.

2. Pick your plants.

After you choose your protein, add your fruit or vegetables. Breakfast might have a fruit, and most lunches and dinners should have at least two large handfuls of leafy green or nonstarchy vegetables. Plants give us fiber, vitamins, and phytochemicals, which are biologically active compounds that include antioxidants, which can help prevent disease. The fiber in plants and whole grains feeds your gut bacteria and increases satiety.

3. Add fat for flavor.

You'll also need some fat to make things satisfying and delicious. Cheese, oil, butter, and avocado are some good examples. Some foods like farmed salmon have fat in them already, but you can also add more to your meal. Like I said earlier, a nourishing diet has a variety of all fats.

4. Add carbs for energy.

As we discussed in the carbs chapter, you might have carbs at every meal, and you might not. If your meal has grain-based carbs or starchy vegetables, start with ½–1 cup (around the size of your fist), and if you don't find that to be enough, bump it up by half a cup at a time. If you want to decrease the amount, do it by half-cup increments.

Not all meals are going to have these things, but most of them should. Not all days are going to have these things, but most of them should. If they don't, don't worry about it. Nutrition doesn't go day by day; it's more of a long game. If your diet is mostly complete and varied with the above things, you should be absolutely fine.

Breakfast

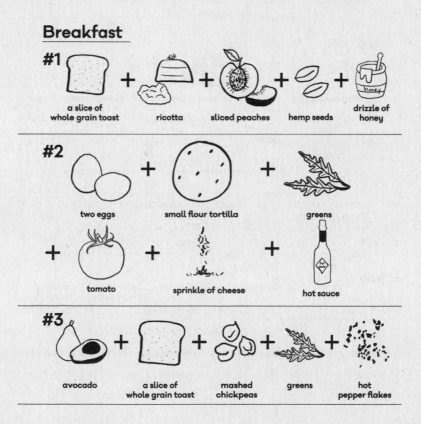

#1

a slice of whole grain toast + ricotta + sliced peaches + hemp seeds + drizzle of honey

#2

two eggs + small flour tortilla + greens + tomato + sprinkle of cheese + hot sauce

#3

avocado + a slice of whole grain toast + mashed chickpeas + greens + hot pepper flakes

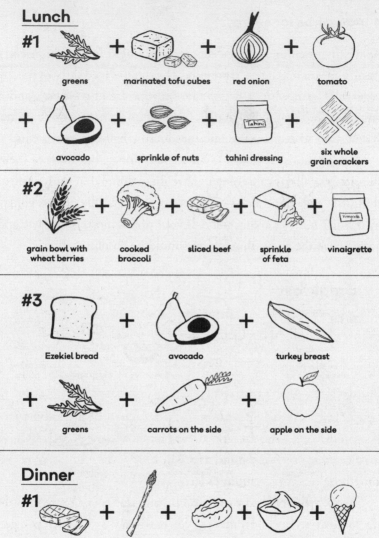

Lunch

#1

greens + marinated tofu cubes + red onion + tomato

+ avocado + sprinkle of nuts + tahini dressing + six whole grain crackers

#2

grain bowl with wheat berries + cooked broccoli + sliced beef + sprinkle of feta + vinaigrette

#3

Ezekiel bread + avocado + turkey breast

+ greens + carrots on the side + apple on the side

Dinner

#1

steak filet + asparagus + baked potato + sour cream on baked potato + scoop of ice cream for dessert

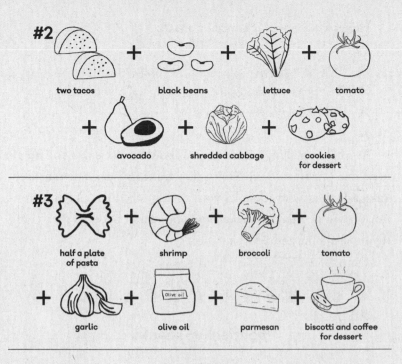

#2

two tacos + black beans + lettuce + tomato

+ avocado + shredded cabbage + cookies for dessert

#3

half a plate of pasta + shrimp + broccoli + tomato

+ garlic + olive oil + parmesan + biscotti and coffee for dessert

SNACKS

So what is a snack, anyway? They're usually about ½–⅓ the size of a meal, for starters. The most nourishing snacks are a combination of protein, carbs, and fat, and they're foods you enjoy because this satisfies your body *and* mind and will keep you from foraging for something else fifteen minutes later.

Snacks aren't generally used to fill your stomach; they're for tiding you over to your next meal so you're not ravenous when you get there. There's a trend now to snack more often and eat fewer meals; I don't recommend doing this for a few reasons: 1) It's easier to eat more when you're grazing all day. 2) If you snack all day, chances are you're not sitting down and eating mindfully. This doesn't signal to your body that you've eaten, and it's more likely that you'll be hunting for something else to eat soon after.

Here's when you might need a snack:

✖ You're going more than around four hours between meals.
✖ You've had a workout and your next meal is hours away.
✖ You're hungry between meals.

As with everything, the takeaway about snacks is that you might need one or two or even three a day, but this is so individualized. Take a look at your lifestyle, your eating schedule, and your routine. Try to be mindful about how you feel in between meals, and if you need one, add a snack.

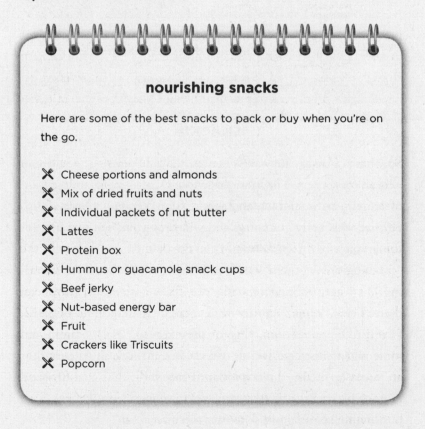

nourishing snacks

Here are some of the best snacks to pack or buy when you're on the go.

✖ Cheese portions and almonds
✖ Mix of dried fruits and nuts
✖ Individual packets of nut butter
✖ Lattes
✖ Protein box
✖ Hummus or guacamole snack cups
✖ Beef jerky
✖ Nut-based energy bar
✖ Fruit
✖ Crackers like Triscuits
✖ Popcorn

SUPPLEMENTS

If you're eating a varied diet, you should be getting everything you need in that. Multivitamins are generally not helpful for most of the population because they contain a lot of what we generally don't need—like many of the B vitamins that are readily available in food. People who may benefit from multivitamins are those who are at risk for several deficiencies and can't eat enough to keep up with their recommended daily intake of vitamins and minerals. It's important to check that the multivitamin you choose has enough of each vitamin and mineral you need to satisfy your daily requirements.

Supplementation isn't a one-size-fits-all situation. We don't all need vitamin D or iron supplements, for example. If you're deficient in one single vitamin or mineral, a multivitamin might not contain enough of it to make a difference, which is why in many cases, I'd recommend supplementing with individual vitamins and minerals according to what you actually need. It's a more targeted approach. For example, if you're a vegan, you may need B12 if you're not eating B12-fortified foods. If you're a woman of childbearing age with heavy periods, you're at risk for having low iron. If you live in a northern climate, you may need vitamin D more than someone who lives in, say, Arizona. But instead of just gulping down supplements because you think you might be deficient in certain vitamins and minerals, the best thing to do is to get tested to see if you're actually low in them.

As we age, we're more at risk for certain vitamin and mineral deficiencies. People over fifty need to watch their levels of B6, B12, vitamin D, and calcium. One of the main causes of vitamin and mineral deficiencies as we age is decreased intake of food overall or an increased intake of ultraprocessed foods. If you're over fifty and don't think your diet is adequate, you may need a supplement. This is something to ask your doctor or dietitian about.

SHOPPING AND COOKING

Now that we know what our meals and snacks should look like, let's talk about how we get that food onto the plate to begin with. Yes, I'm talking about grocery shopping. We touched on this a little in Chapter 4 on mapping your goals, but now it's time to dive in deeper.

Before you shop, choose three proteins for the week. You might want chicken, fish, and chickpeas. Buy the best-quality food you can afford, but remember that cost-effective foods like eggs, dried beans, and lentils are also high-quality whole proteins. Regardless of what you choose, these are what you're going to build your meals around.

When you're at the store, select three to five vegetables to prep with the proteins, like salad greens, carrots, cucumber, and cauliflower. Choose local and in-season produce if you can, but frozen vegetables count as whole foods, too. Remember, organic food doesn't mean healthier.

Select a starch. Rice, baby potatoes, baking potatoes, or pasta are all examples.

To round everything out, think about what you'll need for breakfasts and snacks for the week: bread, nuts and nut butters, eggs, hummus, fruits (two to three types), and dairy like milk, cheese, and yogurt.

After you do your shopping, batch-cook.

- ✕ Prepare your proteins. Roast your chicken. Bake or panfry your fish. Do a curried chickpea dish. Keep it simple!
- ✕ Prep your vegetables by steaming or roasting some, peeling and cutting others and keeping them raw, whatever way you want to do them.
- ✕ Prep your starch by precooking grains or roasting potatoes. (Except for baked potatoes, which you can microwave when

you want them, and pasta because it's pretty quick and super easy to boil.)

You now have the building blocks for different meals. These blocks can be arranged however you like: You can use the chicken as a main course with vegetables and starch. Or, you could put it into a salad or pasta or quesadillas. I personally love combining chicken with barbecue sauce and stuffing it into baked potatoes with some sort of steamed or sautéed green. Easy. Or at least, not as onerous as you might think. If you're stuck for recipes or just don't feel confident in the kitchen, your best bet would be to take a look at one of the thousands of websites—including my own!—and cookbooks that are dedicated to easy, wholesome cooking, batch cooking, and meal prep. Remember, a diet with variety ensures you're getting all the nutrients your body needs—it's also emotionally satisfying—so don't be afraid to try a new food each week or cook an old favorite in a different way.

At the end of the day, high-value eating should work for you; it should add to your life, not take away. Yes, it means being flexible, keeping things simple, and getting comfortable in the kitchen if you aren't already. It means thinking ahead and prepping the foods and meals you love so you're ready to take on the week. Some weeks, you'll be more successful at all of this than others, but as long as you continue to see the value in high-value eating and make the effort to put it into practice as much as you can, you'll reap the benefits. You'll be emotionally and physically free. You'll save money. You'll be nourishing your body the way it deserves to be nourished. And, you'll be able to eat without guilt, shame, anxiety, or restriction. Win-win-win.

gut health

No, I'm not talking about intuition. I'm talking about the health of the bacteria that live in our intestines, metabolize our food, and so much more. Why? you ask. Well, you can follow all the steps I've laid out for you to nourish your body properly, but if you don't consider your gut health, you're missing a key piece of the puzzle.

Our microbiome, which is the population of bacteria (microbiota) in our gut, is thought to influence everything from our mood to our immunity. Seventy to 80 percent of our immune system is in our gut.[1] The microbiota also help digest food, especially carbohydrates, break down toxins and medications, control inflammation, and may impact how our genes express themselves (the delivery of information from DNA to the genes to create molecules like proteins). This is important because the way a gene is expressed can affect our health and our risk for disease, although we aren't yet sure exactly how our gut bacteria does this.

There is also some discussion about whether our microbiome has an effect on our weight, and we suspect that it does in some way. Many believe that we metabolize food and absorb calories differently according to our gut-bacteria profiles. However, that's basically all we know: We're not at the point where you can switch up your gut bacteria to optimize weight loss. All you can do is make sure that your little gut bugs are happy; this is the best way to improve your overall health.

Sleep and stress go hand in hand with gut health. Not only are they absolutely linked to what we choose to eat, as we've touched on earlier, but they also affect how we metabolize our food. Gut health, sleep, and stress are like the icing on the nourishing diet cake—they're not everything, but they finish it all off and are definitely an important ingredient. In fact, few things impact our nutrition and health like our guts, sleep patterns, and stress levels. In this chapter, I'm going to walk you through the integral role all three play on our health so you can function at your very best.

Let's start with our gut.

WHAT IS OUR GUT?

Our gut—otherwise known as our intestinal tract, is home to one of the largest colonies of bacteria in our body: our microbiome. The microbiome is even considered by some to be another organ in our bodies and the total weight of it can be up to 2 kg.[2] That's almost five pounds of bacteria. Yeah, the thought of that makes me squirm, too.

Each of us has our own gut microbiota profile. While we share the same 1,000 gut-bacteria species, your profile will be different than everyone else's, thanks to what you eat, how you live, and where you live. People in different parts of the world have vastly different gut microbiota, tailored to digesting the host's native diet.[3,4]

So, how do these little guys work?

Think of your gut as a fermenting tank. When we eat food that contains fermentable fiber—otherwise known as *prebiotics*—such as the fiber in legumes, oats, fruits, root vegetables, and nuts, it travels to our large intestine, where it's broken down and fermented by our gut bacteria.[5] This process nourishes the bacteria while producing short-chain fatty acids (SCFAs) called butyrate, proprionate, and acetate, which help provide energy to cells in the colon, balance blood sugar, reduce inflammation, protect the colonic cells, and may even destroy cancer cells in the colon.[6] All good stuff!

But if we eat a diet that's very high in protein and low in fiber, that fermentation process results in different compounds that can swing the microbiome balance in favor of pathogenic bacteria, which are damaging to our health.[7] This may cause inflammation and a higher risk for conditions such as colon cancer, inflammatory bowel disease, diabetes, and even fatty liver. The consumption of a diet high in fiber can control this effect. In other words, fiber is our gut's best friend.

While eating fiber goes a long way to ensuring good gut health, a less-than-ideal diet, stress, travel, illness, and antibiotics, among other things, can cause dysbiosis, which is when there is an imbalance in your gut bacteria—either there has been a die-off of good bacteria, an overgrowth of pathogenic bacteria, or a loss of diversity overall. The repercussions are not fun. Symptoms can include diarrhea, bloating, gas, and constipation. Dysbiosis can affect your immune system, making you more susceptible to pathogens and infection. It's also implicated in conditions such as obesity, inflammatory bowel disease, and allergies; whether dysbiosis is a cause or an effect of these conditions we don't know, as microbiome research is in its infancy.[8] Still, it's widely accepted that keeping our microbiome healthy and diverse is important for our health. And diet, sleep, and stress all play a huge role in that.

Let's start with how what we eat affects our gut.

PREBIOTICS AND PROBIOTICS

When I talk about nutrition and gut health, prebiotics and probiotics are usually one of the first things people want to know about. As we discussed above, *prebiotics* are the fiber that feeds your gut bacteria. *Probiotics* are the actual good bacteria that live in your gut. The official definition of a probiotic is live microorganisms that, when taken in adequate amounts, confer a health benefit on the host.[9] In other words, when you eat enough probiotics, you're populating your gut with more of the good guys.

The plant-forward eating habits that you've learned so far in this book are already gut-friendly, but there are other good-for-the-gut foods you can add to your diet. Some prebiotic-rich foods are:

- bananas
- oats
- Jerusalem artichokes
- legumes
- onions
- leeks
- garlic
- asparagus[10]

Probiotic foods include fermented options such as:

- ✕ miso
- ✕ tempeh
- ✕ sauerkraut
- ✕ kimchi
- ✕ yogurt
- ✕ kefir

But not all of these contain the right bugs, in the right amounts, every time we eat them. This is one of the challenges of probiotic foods.

For example, most of us have heard that yogurt is a good source of probiotics. My mother used to force yogurt on me whenever I took antibiotics as a kid, which was a lot! In reality, not every yogurt is probiotic. Some have probiotics, but those don't survive their trip through the stomach to the intestine, where they ferment. And even if they do, recent research shows that the levels in the product are often too low to have any effect.[11] While some yogurts claim to help fight colds, lower cholesterol, decrease cavities, and improve IBS symptoms, the above study found that you'd have to eat up to twenty-five servings of some yogurts to get these effects. Thanks, but no thanks. I'd rather just live with my cold. Yogurt and other products can also be full of sugar, which negates the point of eating them for their probiotics, in my opinion.

There are also different strains of probiotics that do different things in different amounts, which is important if you're selecting a probiotic for a specific issue—like bloating or diarrhea, or just for general health. But when it comes to food, we just don't know the amount and strains of probiotics that these foods contain, and it's not enough to have the vague claim of probiotics on the label. It's all fine to claim that your tortilla chips have probiotics in them, but which probiotic bacteria do they contain and how much? Are they going to make it past your stomach acid? That information is probably not available, and it's all too common for people to be swayed by the claim without having all the necessary facts. In truth, there's no real evidence that foods that have added probiotics in them (hello, probiotic chocolate) have any positive effects on our health.

Fermented foods like kimchi and sauerkraut don't have a probiotic claim on their labels, and sometimes they're not even labeled: The Polish deli near my brother's house has a barrel of sauerkraut in the back, which is how it's sold. That stuff is probably probiotic AF, but nobody will ever know for sure. Other fermented foods that naturally contain probiotics are kefir, tempeh, miso, and kombucha (watch the sugar content in this!).

There's no harm in adding probiotic foods to your diet, and I think that fermented foods, as opposed to foods that have added probiotics are your best bet. Remember, though, that the organisms in the product need to be live to be considered probiotic.[12] Look for products that say "naturally fermented" and contain bubbles in the jar, which indicate the presence of live bacteria. Don't cook them, since heat will destroy their good bacteria.

If you need a probiotic, supplements are the best way to get the right amounts and strains, though the research is mixed. Some studies suggest that certain probiotics may reduce frequency and duration of the common cold and help alleviate IBS symptoms, but many are conflictive or inconclusive, or don't have solid methodology.[13,14] Some people do find probiotics helpful, especially for conditions that have positive research behind their use—mostly antibiotic-induced diarrhea and C-difficile. However, in most cases, we don't know how much of which probiotic to take to effectively treat different ailments.

That being said, probiotic supplements are generally safe, so if you have gut issues and want to try them, ask your pharmacist for their recommendations. Here are a few things to remember.

- ✖ The probiotic in the supplement works in the large intestine, not in the stomach. This means that the probiotic itself has to be encapsulated in a way that prevents it from getting destroyed in the acidic environment of the stomach. Make sure the probiotic you're buying specifically states that it can move through the stomach unharmed.
- ✖ The two most common probiotic bacteria are Lactobacillus and Bifidobacterium.
- ✖ More bugs aren't always better. I'm guilty of this, too—most of us want to choose the probiotic that has the most bacteria, usually something like 50 billion CFU (colony-forming units). But what's more important is buying the correct strain for what you need it for and making sure the probiotic is fresh, since they do expire.

While the FDA has not approved any probiotic to treat illness, some companies have taken the time to do thorough research on their product. I feel like in the future we'll each have a prescribed personal probiotic strain that matches our microbiome. Unfortunately, the science to do that isn't there yet. In the meantime, talk to your pharmacist for a recommendation to get the best product for your concerns.

myth buster:

gut-bacteria test kits.

You can now get gut-bacteria test kits that come with diet and nutrition advice tailored to your personal microbiome. While this sounds very forward-thinking, the common consensus from the scientific community (and myself) is that the science isn't there yet. We can get our microbiome read, but we don't know what to do with that information, especially when it comes to making recommendations for weight loss. Since there's no value in getting information that we don't know how to interpret yet, I'd pass on these tests for now.

SLEEP PATTERNS

When I sit down with clients for the first time, I ask them all sorts of questions that don't seem to pertain to nutrition, like how they're sleeping and if they have a stressful life. They sort of look at me funny, like "I thought this was about nutrition?" and then I explain that things like sleep and stress are absolutely linked to our diets and our gut health.

Sleep and nutrition are a two-way street. Lack of sleep affects our food choices, but our food choices can also affect the quality of our sleep.[15]

My mom used to tell me that I wouldn't grow if I didn't sleep. Nice scare tactic, Mom! But she was partly correct: Sleep influences the release of growth hormones. It also impacts glucose tolerance

and plays into the release of cortisol, leptin, and ghrelin, all hormones that you're familiar with by now.[16] Studies suggest that sleep
debt increases insulin resistance as well as levels of ghrelin and cortisol, and decreases leptin—and this is likely in part why lack of
sleep has been linked to obesity.[17] When your leptin is low and your
ghrelin is high, it's tough to stop eating. It's just science.

Sleep deprivation also affects our endocannabinoid system (ECS).
Unlike the cannabinoids in marijuana, endocannabinoids are lipid-
based neurotransmitters made by your body that help to regulate
appetite, among other functions. While research on the ECS is just
ramping up—it was discovered in the 1990s—early studies indicate
that inadequate sleep may increase the amount of endocannabinoids
in your blood, and thus a desire to eat.[18] This is what happens when
you smoke or consume marijuana and get the "munchies," except in
that case, cannabinoids, not *endo*cannabinoids, are to blame.

Beyond these chemical reactions taking place in your body,
sleep deprivation also causes physical exhaustion, which means you
may not have the energy or desire to be active or to prepare your
own meals. You may also gravitate toward comfort foods to sort of
"cocoon" yourself in to make yourself feel better. Being on a diet
that's too low in carbs or very high in refined carbs may also cause
sleep disturbance.[19]

Sometimes, getting enough sleep and dialing down the stress in
our lives is harder than it looks. As a parent, I know how aggravat-
ing it can be to hear how we need eight hours of sleep a day, that
sleep heals everything, and that sleep deprivation is detrimental to
health. When my kids were really young and kept me up all night,
I wanted to throw my computer against the wall every time I saw
some celebrity pontificating about the importance of getting your
beauty sleep. I wanted to sleep more than you could ever imagine,
but I couldn't control my kids waking me up in the middle of the

night. Any of you parents know exactly what I'm talking about. The average adult gets around seven hours of sleep a night, but clearly, they didn't survey new parents, or insomniacs, for this figure.

Being up all night with kids is one thing, but many of us are sleep deprived by choice. Meaning, we don't prioritize sleep like we should. Instead, we sit on our smartphones all night, binge-watch Netflix into the wee hours, or work into the early hours. In our busy, hectic lives, sleep often gets shoved onto the back burner. We think we'll make up our sleep debt on the weekend or when we're on vacation, but face it, that rarely happens. When it does, it's never enough. We're just too busy, and we can't shut our brains off.

By this point in the book you know that my MO is: Do your best. It's also: Don't try to control everything. And that applies to sleep, too. You might not be able to control your kid waking you up in the middle of the night, but you can definitely try to improve your sleep through your habits and your diet.

For some of us, going to bed at a reasonable time and getting a solid night's sleep is pretty much impossible, at least consistently. Whatever the cause, try to optimize your time in bed as much as you can. If you know you're probably going to be woken up in the middle of the night, try to hit the sack a bit earlier to front-load your sleep. Leave the dishes and the laundry, and get your ass to bed. You know the drill:

- ✖ Don't watch TV or use your smartphone in bed before you sleep like my husband does. (Yes, I yell at him to stop.)
- ✖ Keep the same sleep schedule as much as possible, even on weekends.
- ✖ Keep your bedroom cool.
- ✖ Write down whatever you're worried about if it's keeping you awake.

These small habitual changes will improve what's called your sleep hygiene. But it's also important that you eat for sleep. Read on.

MELATONIN

Melatonin is a neurohormone our brains make that regulates sleep, but it can also be found in some foods, which when eaten before bedtime can help you fall asleep faster. Melatonin-rich foods include: tart cherries, bananas, pineapples, almonds, walnuts, and oats.[20,21] You can also take melatonin supplements, but as I always say, try to get what you need from food first.

TRYPTOPHAN

This is an amino acid found in dairy, meats, and seeds. Maybe you've heard that turkey and milk make us tired because they contain tryptophan. Tryptophan is a precursor to melatonin, meaning our bodies use tryptophan to produce melatonin. It's also used to make serotonin, famously known for being the neurotransmitter that relaxes us.[22]

When we eat tryptophan-rich foods, their tryptophan is converted in the brain to the compound 5-HTP (5-hydroxytryptophan), then to serotonin, then to melatonin. This doesn't mean you should take serotonin supplements. It's all about the tryptophan, which can cross the blood-brain barrier, unlike serotonin. And while 5-HTP supplements exist, the evidence that they aid in sleep is inconclusive. There is no official dosage of 5-HTP for sleep, and the quality of supplements can vary. Most importantly, 5-HTP taken in conjunction with some other medications—especially SSRIs—can be lethal.

MAGNESIUM

Magnesium is an element that helps our bodies maintain nerve and muscle function, keeps bones strong, and supports our immune system.[23] It also increases GABA (gamma aminobutyric acid), a neurotransmitter that helps us relax. In other words, it's good for sleep and our guts.

However, a high percentage of U.S. adults don't get the recommended 320–420 mg of magnesium in their daily diets.[24] People with GI conditions that cause chronic diarrhea and malabsorption such as Crohn's disease or celiac disease; alcoholics; people with type 2 diabetes; people with a low-magnesium diet, and older adults are all at risk for magnesium deficiency.

The good news is that magnesium is readily available in our food. The best food sources are almonds, cashews, peanuts and peanut butter, spinach, black beans, edamame, and whole wheat bread.

There are also magnesium supplements that you can take before bedtime to help with sleep. Choose one that dissolves in water for maximum absorbency. Magnesium citrate is a good option that's commonly used in sleep-promoting magnesium supplements. Remember that magnesium is also a laxative (hence milk of magnesia), so take it according to package directions.

ALCOHOL

Booze might be good at putting you into a deep sleep. Alcohol increases our production of adenosine, which is a compound that induces sleep. That's good enough to make you tired and get you into bed, but that's not the end of the story, sleepwise.

When you have more than one drink, your brain shows a lot of *delta* activity, or slow-wave sleep. This is deep restful sleep that you'll experience for the first half of the night. That's all good, except that after we drink, *alpha* activity, which normally happens when you're relaxed but not asleep, steps in later on. The alpha and delta activity together inhibit deep sleep, making you feel unrested when you wake up.

Alcohol also tends to reduce REM sleep, the sleep stage in which you dream.[25] It's the most restorative sleep stage, which again explains why you feel like you didn't even sleep when you wake up after a night of drinking.

And ever wonder why after you drink, you're up at the crack of dawn? That's because by that time, your body has had the chance to metabolize the booze you guzzled the night before and the sleep-promoting chemical adenosine that got you into bed in the first place has now worn off. Worst feeling ever.

STRESS LEVELS

Stress and sleep are related, and so are stress and nutrition. Stress affects our ability to sleep, which can lead to overeating. But it can also affect the balance of our gut bacteria.[26, 27, 28]

As we talked about before, the type and diversity of the bacteria in our gut can directly affect our health. Even though research on how stress affects gut bacteria is still in its early stages, there are studies that suggest that prolonged stress can affect intestinal permeability, which may lead to inflammation in our body. This may be why when we're stressed, we're more prone to flare-ups of IBS and other conditions.

Stress affects the chemistry of our bodies and it all leads back to cortisol. Remember the flight or fight response we discussed in the carb chapter? Here's a reminder. When we're stressed, our body needs more energy to fight the perceived threat, so it releases cortisol, which increases our appetite and suppresses our insulin production.[29] Insulin helps control the amount of sugar in the blood, but our body wants that sugar for energy. As if that isn't enough, elevated cortisol levels also tell our body to release triglycerides for energy, which can cause high triglyceride levels in the blood. In cases of chronic stress, the fight-or-flight instinct is constant, resulting in increased hunger, weight gain, and a buildup of sugar and triglycerides in the blood, which may lead to type 2 diabetes and elevated risk of heart disease.

We're not done with cortisol yet, that naughty monkey. High levels of cortisol suppress our immune system, leaving us susceptible to illness. That feeling of being run-down when you're burning the candle at both ends? It's a real thing. Cortisol also compromises our GI system in order to save energy. But when digestion slows, we experience bloating, constipation, and eventually malabsorption and inflammation. It makes you wonder how many people with IBS symptoms are suffering from chronic stress! But if you have IBS or IBD, you might also notice that stress triggers your symptoms and flare-ups. That's because of cortisol.

In terms of food choices, when we're stressing about something, sometimes we feel like we need crunchy, fatty, or sugary foods to ease our mood. It goes back to emotional eating. When we're stressed or unhappy we tend to choose foods that transport us back to simpler, happier times. This can mean your favorite childhood birthday dessert or whatever food you associate with being stress-free and content. It can also mean that when we're angry or stressed, we crave crunchy food because we want to kick the shit out of something. Make sense?

But that's not the only reason we crave comfort foods when we're stressed. Recent research suggests that in some people, eating sugary, fatty foods in response to stress may decrease the body's hypothalmic pituitary adrenal axis stress response in the long-term.[30, 31] Meaning, people who chronically self-medicate their stress with food may actually be decreasing all that cortisol and hormone secretion. Unfortunately, the other side of the coin is greater abdominal obesity, which is detrimental to health.

Certain diets also cause us more stress. Hell, dieting itself causes stress! When you're constantly worried about what you can and can't eat, how much you weigh, and whether you're going to feel obligated to share a platter of chicken wings with your workmates on Thirsty Thursday, that shit gets stressful. And if you happen to be cutting carbs, things get even worse because very low-carb diets (10 percent of calories or less) are associated with elevated levels of cortisol, so without adequate carbs, your body is in a state of low-level stress.[32] All. The. Time. That can't be healthy, right? Yeah, it's not.

Okay, so now that I've thoroughly exhausted you, here are some things you can do:

- ✂ Decrease stress in your life any way you can.
- ✂ Don't diet. (You know that already.)
- ✂ Don't cut carbs to the point where you're miserable, deprived, and stressed out.
- ✂ Eat to help your stress.

If you have a lot of stress that you can't reduce with lifestyle changes, you should be eating foods that reduce inflammation. High-value eating is already anti-inflammatory: it contains lots of whole foods, fruits and vegetables, whole grains, and less sugar and ultraprocessed items. Avoiding trans and high levels of saturated fats is also important for keeping inflammation at bay. Caffeinated beverages such as coffee have been known to increase stress levels, so avoid adding insult to injury by cutting down caffeine when you're overly stressed.

There are a lot of articles online that tout the cortisol-reducing powers of B and C vitamins, but the truth is that research either doesn't support or is conflicted about these theories. While magnesium might be good for sleep, there are no studies that encourage its use in cortisol reduction. Some research suggests using DHA to lower cortisol, but the studies are low quality and the results aren't convincing.

Interestingly, what does appear to lower cortisol levels in humans is ashwangandha, an adaptogen that's derived from a plant in the nightshade family (flowering plants like tomatoes, eggplant, and peppers).[33, 34] If you decide to take an ashwangandha supplement, consult your pharmacist to cross-reference it with any other medications you may be taking. Ashwangandha is known to interact with thyroid medications, steroids, and sedatives, among others.

You may never have guessed how much our gut, sleep patterns, and stress levels ripple out to affect our diet. But keeping them all in check and optimizing them to the best of your ability can have a profound effect on your mood, food, and overall wellness.

If you follow the high-value eating plan, prioritize your right to rest, and say no to some of the stuff that makes your life crazy, you'll be naturally helping your gut, sleep, and stress levels. Those are the key ingredients in a recipe for success.

conclusion:
moving forward

We've been on quite the journey together. We've talked about diet culture and how harmful and insidious it is. We discussed the shitty things we say to ourselves, why we repeat them over and over, and how that affects us. We pulled out those negative core values of ours, turned them over in our hands, and told them to get lost. We did a few science lessons about macronutrients and what your body needs to be happy and healthy. Then we talked about how to put those lessons into practice and how to care for yourself in other ways, namely getting more sleep and knocking down the stress. We did it!

So what now? If you haven't already, you can start to put what we learned into practice. As you move forward, here are some key points to remember.

Living your best life means grabbing life by the balls and being in the present, instead of wallowing in the toxic garbage pile of diet culture. Instead of giving such a crap about what celebrities and influencers are eating and how much they weigh, put the focus on the things that matter most to you and the people you love. When you do the opposite—focus on numbers, counting, weight, what you can and can't eat, and how you want to fit into your jeans from twenty years ago—it costs you. It costs you financially because you're buying into diets and products that are bogus. It costs you physically because it's exhausting and unhealthy to gain and lose the same weight over and over again. And it costs you emotionally because you feel guilty and sad about not achieving the unrealistic goals that diet culture sets out for you. Those costs are far too high. Let them go. It may be a trade-off—some extra pounds for a lifetime of freedom from diets, but isn't that worth it?

Understand that diets and the wellness industry are big business, and our society feeds into that. They don't exist for your health; they exist to make money off unsuspecting people.

It's hard to get away from all of the noise, but one way is to unfollow anyone online who makes you feel bad about yourself. Comparing yourself to other people is normal human behavior, but it's a lesson in futility, especially on social media. There are a lot of unknowns behind those pretty pictures, and chances are, you're being misled.

Even outside of social media, remember that your genetics, lifestyle, socioeconomic status, likes and dislikes, and upbringing are unique. Spending your life wanting what someone else has when it may or may not be attainable to you is a waste of time that could otherwise be spent bringing joy to yourself and others. Find your own strengths and revel in them.

YOU FIT INTO THIS WORLD THE WAY YOU ARE. Don't be afraid to take up space. In fact, go out there and take up all the space you need. When you reject the box that others want to put you into, you set an example for everyone else. From one disruptor to another, just do it.

Find your core beliefs. This is something that we rarely think of doing. Most of us don't even know how deeply these beliefs affect our choices through our lives. The core beliefs that are negative can be a major stumbling block to living in the present. Remember that boulder that rolls down the hill and lands on top of you, again and again, not letting you get to where you want to go? Time to slingshot that boulder into oblivion by taking a long, hard look at why it's there. Ask yourself "why" and go back to Chapter 2 and do this work as many times as you need to; this is the key to making changes to your eating and lifestyle and sustaining them well into the future. If you need help from a therapist to guide you, please get it. Because once you trash those beliefs by asking yourself the hard questions, you open yourself to a life unfettered by guilt, shame, and anxiety around food and eating. One in which you can move forward being who you are and own what's rightfully yours: happiness and freedom with food and your body.

Normal eating is a huge spectrum. Understanding that can change how you feel about your food choices. Overeating sometimes? Normal. Feeling hungry all the time because of food restriction? Not normal. The list of normal eating habits in Chapter 3 is there to remind you that food and eating should be flexible, fun, and free of negative emotion.

Trust your body. It isn't going to end in disaster. Remember the hunger and fullness scale and use it to find your true hunger.

Set realistic goals. Focus on your comfortable weight, not a number on the scale. Don't be afraid to readjust if it's not working.

Carbs aren't harmful. Protein helps with physical satisfaction. Fat isn't anything to be afraid of. Water is best, but coffee counts, too. Don't get bogged down by the numbers. We don't eat ingredients in isolation; we eat food. Variety of diet is the key to true nourishment; if you do that, you'll get all the nutrients you need.

Be a pencil, not an eraser. It's important to add food to your diet, not take it away. Know your hunger, lifestyle, and preferences, and be balanced, flexible, and intentional—because goddamn it, you're going to eat that brownie and move the fuck on with life. Yes, you'll have to make some changes; this is the key to sustainable change. It takes some time to adjust certain habits. Do the best you can and don't beat yourself up. Eat the way YOU want, not for anyone else. If you don't do this for you, you shouldn't do it at all.

And finally, if there's one message you take away from this book, it's that all food is good and all diets are bad. The reason food exists is to nourish us physically, though its purpose goes beyond that. Food brings us together and nourishes us emotionally. It tells the stories of our cultures. It delights us and fills us with joy. Those are all good things that we all have a right to enjoy. Exercise that right. This leads to true satisfaction.

So here we are at the end. I hope you feel empowered as you move forward.

Thank you for trusting me to impart what I've learned to you. Thank you for taking the time to read this book, and for integrating my knowledge into your life and your habits. Thank you for allowing me to change the way you think about food, eating, and your body.

It has been a privilege to work with you.

abby XO

acknowledgments

Getting a book deal is all fun and games . . . until you realize that you then have to actually write a book . . . which has to be the most perfect 65,000 words you've ever written. Yeah, there's that. So it's important that I thank everyone who has helped me on this massive journey.

This book is dedicated to my family: Ryan, Jordan, and Isabel, who have supported me with a minimum (most of the time) of whining while I not only built Abby Langer Nutrition as a business, but also as I wrote this book all day long, and on vacations, weekends, and holidays. Writing a book takes forever, but my family has always given me unconditional love in spite of it all. And to Sammy, my furry, four-legged son, thanks for keeping me company while I was writing and for keeping me warm with your snuggles. I love you guys.

There are a lot of other people who have been with me on this crazy journey. My mom, who is my best friend, my rock, and who always keeps me grounded and sane, even when shit goes sideways. She always counsels me to stop, breathe, and take another look at things. We all need someone like that in our lives, and I'm so lucky to have her.

My dad, who's in heaven, from whom I inherited a brain for science and a drive to disrupt. He was a maverick surgeon who taught me not to let what other people think of me stand in the way of doing what I believe is right. Your light still shines so bright, Dad. Oh, and thank you for the dimes. I love you and miss you, too.

My mother-in-law, Deb Swain, who's always ready to come over with some meat loaf and mashed potatoes, or to help with the kids and the dog while I work. And she always wipes my kitchen counters so they sparkle before she leaves our house, so I don't have to. You're the mother-in-law from central casting. Thank you.

My brother, Eli, and his wife, Jen, who are always there to support me. I love you both.

Desiree Neilson, RD, my friend and author of *Eat More Plants*, who listened patiently to my book idea in a dark restaurant all those months ago, encouraged me to write it, and generously introduced me to her superstar agent, Carly Watters at P.S. Literary. Thank you Desiree, because you believed in me, and without you, this book might not exist.

Carly Watters, my agent, what can I say. I know that helping me write my book proposal was like trying to get blood from a stone, but somehow you managed without giving up on me. Trust me, there were a few points in that process when I thought that's where the conversation was going to go. You've always had my back, you ferocious mama bear, and I am so grateful to have you on my side. Thank you.

Thank you to Simon & Schuster Canada, who took a chance on me as a first-time author, even though I walked into our first meeting reeking of the skunk that had sprayed my dog less than an hour before. Best icebreaker ever! And Sarah St. Pierre, my editor, you're a rock star for wading through my clunky AF first draft like an absolute champ, rearranging and editing and cutting and fluffing. You deserve a medal, or at least a really long vacation, for all of that heavy lifting. Thank you for your tireless work in making this book something I am so very proud of.

My badass dietitian posse, including Cara Rosenbloom, Nicole Osinga, Laura Baum, Christy Wilson, Abbey Sharp, Amanda Hamel, and everyone else who listened to me bitch about trolls, work, and everything else, and who also answered my sometimes very annoying and technical questions while I wrote this book. I'm so thankful for colleagues like you, who are generous, kind, and always ready to listen.

To my other friends, my Dal buddies, the girls in my neighborhood, my bestie Kathryn Weiser, my California ladies, I love you all. Thank you so much for your friendship and support.

To my followers who have been dedicated and supportive and such cheerleaders this entire way. Thank you so much for reading my stuff, for your wonderful comments, and for knowing the value of a good rant with an f-bomb or two.

And lastly, to my haters, you know who you are. I know you might not want to believe this, but as my dad would say, you've done me a big favor. Your mean and nasty comments kept me grounded, and gave me even more motivation to write this book and get my message out into the world.

And here we are.

notes

chapter 1: ditch the diet

1. Global Wellness Institute, "Wellness Industry Statistics & Facts," *Global Wellness Institute*, October 2018, https://globalwellnessinstitute.org/pressroom/statistics-and-facts/.

2. C. C. Simpson and S. E. Mazzeo, "Skinny Is Not Enough: A Content Analysis of Fitspiration on Pinterest," *Health Commun* 32, no. 5 (2017): 560–567, doi:10.1080/10410236.2016.1140273.

3. European Association for the Study of Obesity, "Study scrutinizes credibility of weight management blogs by most popular influencers on social media," *EurekAlert!*, April 29, 2019, https://www.eurekalert.org/pub_releases/2019-04/eaft-ssc042919.php.

4. Mary Sherlock and Danielle Wagstaff, "Exploring the Relationship Between Frequency of Instagram Use, Exposure to Idealized Images, and Psychological Well-Being in Women," *Psychology of Popular Media* 8, no. 4 (2019), 482–90, doi:10.1037/ppm0000182.

5. Grace Holland and Marika Tiggemann, "A systematic review of the impact of the use of social networking sites on body image and disordered eating outcomes," *Body Image* 17 (2016): 100–11, doi:10.1016/j.bodyim.2016.02.008.

chapter 3: know your hunger

1. A. J. Hill, "The psychology of food craving: Symposium on 'Molecular mechanisms and psychology of food intake,'" *Proceedings of the Nutrition Society* 66, no. 2 (2007): 277–85, doi:10.1017/S0029665107005502.
2. A. Massey and A. J. Hill, "Dieting and food craving. A descriptive, quasi-prospective study," *Appetite* 58, no. 3 (2012): 781–85, doi:10.1016/j.appet.2012.01.020.
3. A. J. Hill, "The psychology of food craving," *Proc Nutr Soc.* 66, no. 2 (May 2007): 277–85, doi:10.1017/S0029665107005502.
4. J. Alcock, C. C. Maley, and C. A. Aktipi, "Is eating behavior manipulated by the gastrointestinal microbiota? Evolutionary pressures and potential mechanisms," *Bioessays* 36, no. 10 (2014): 940–49, doi:10.1002/bies.201400071.

chapter 5: #carbsarelife

1. M. A. Stephens and G. Wand, "Stress and the HPA axis: role of glucocorticoids in alcohol dependence," *Alcohol Res.* 34, no. 4 (2012): 468–83.
2. C. D. Gardner, J. F. Trepanowski, L. C. Del Gobbo, et al, "Effect of Low-Fat vs Low-Carbohydrate Diet on 12-Month Weight Loss in Overweight Adults and the Association with Genotype Pattern or Insulin Secretion: The DIETFITS Randomized Clinical Trial," *JAMA* 319, no. 7 (2018): 667–79, doi:10.1001/jama.2018.0245.
3. L. Thau, J. Gandhi, and S. Sharma, "Physiology, Cortisol," *StatPearls Publishing* (May 2020), https://www.ncbi.nlm.nih.gov/books/NBK538239/.
4. D. S. Ludwig and C. B. Ebbeling, "The Carbohydrate-Insulin Model of Obesity: Beyond 'Calories In, Calories Out,'" *JAMA Intern Med.* 178, no. 8 (2018): 1098–103, doi:10.1001/jamainternmed.2018.2933.
5. Kevin D. Hall, Thomas Bemis, Robert Brychta, Kong Y. Chen, et al, "Calorie for Calorie, Dietary Fat Restriction Results in More Body Fat Loss Than Carbohydrate Restriction in People with Obesity," *Cell Metabolism* 22, no. 3 (2015): 427–36, doi:10.1016/j.cmet.2015.07.021.

chapter 6: prioritize protein

1. M. C. Mojtahedi, M. P. Thorpe, D. C. Karampinos, et al, "The effects of a higher protein intake during energy restriction on changes in body composition and physical function in older women," *Journals of Gerontology: Series A*, 66, no. 11 (2011): 1218–25, doi:10.1093/gerona/glr120.

2. Brian Lindshield, *Kansas State University Human Nutrition Flexbook* (Manhattan: New Prairie Press: 2018), 2.25, https://newprairiepress.org/ebooks/19.

3. Institute of Medicine of the National Academies, *Dietary Reference Intakes for Energy, Carbohydrate, Fiber, Fat, Fatty Acids, Cholesterol, Protein, and Amino Acids* (Washington: National Academies Press, 2005), 691, doi:10.17226/10490.

4. L. Tappy, "Thermic effect of food and sympathetic nervous system activity in humans," *Reprod Nutr Dev.* 36, no. 4 (1996): 391–97, doi:10.1051/rnd:19960405.

5. Jaapna Dhillon, et al, "The Effects of Increased Protein Intake on Fullness: A Meta-Analysis and Its Limitations," *Journal of the Academy of Nutrition and Dietetics* 116, no. 6, 968–83, doi:10.1016/j.jand.2016.01.003.

6. M. Journel, C. Chaumontet, N. Darcel, G. Fromentin, and D. Tomé, "Brain responses to high-protein diets," *Adv Nutr.* 3, no. 3 (May 2012): 322–29, doi:10.3945/an.112.002071.

7. E. Parvaresh Rizi, T. P. Loh, S. Baig, V. Chhay, S. Huang, et al, "A high carbohydrate, but not fat or protein meal attenuates postprandial ghrelin, PYY and GLP-1 responses in Chinese men," *PLoS ONE* 13, no. 1 (2018): e0191609, doi:10.1371/journal.pone.0191609.

8. Douglas Paddon-Jones, Eric Westman, Richard D. Mattes, Robert R. Wolfe, et al, "Protein, weight management, and satiety," *The American Journal of Clinical Nutrition* 87, no. 5 (2008): 1558S–61S, doi:10.1093/ajcn/87.5.1558S.

9. C. M. Hill and C. D. Morrison, "The Protein Leverage Hypothesis: A 2019 Update for *Obesity*," *Obesity* 27, no. 8 (2019): 1221, doi:10.1002/oby.22568.

10. Gertjan Schaafsma, "The Protein Digestibility–Corrected Amino Acid Score," *The Journal of Nutrition* 130, no. 7 (2000): 1865S–67S, doi:10.1093/jn/130.7.1865S.

11. B. J. Schoenfeld and A. A. Aragon, "How much protein can the body use

in a single meal for muscle-building? Implications for daily protein distribution," *Journal of the International Society of Sports Nutrition* 15, no. 10 (2018), doi:10.1186/s12970-018-0215-1.

12. Ann C. Skulas-Ray, Peter W. F. Wilson, William S. Harris, Eliot A. Brinton, et al, "Omega-3 Fatty Acids for the Management of Hypertriglyceridemia: A Science Advisory from the American Heart Association," *Circulation* 140, no. 12 (2019): e673–91, doi:10.1161/CIR.0000000000000709.

13. T. Aung, J. Halsey, D. Kromhout, et al, "Associations of Omega-3 Fatty Acid Supplement Use With Cardiovascular Disease Risks: Meta-analysis of 10 Trials Involving 77917 Individuals," *JAMA Cardiology* 3, no. 3 (2018): 225–34, doi:10.1001/jamacardio.2017.5205.

14. A. S. Abdelhamid, T. J. Brown, J. S. Brainard, et al, "Omega-3 fatty acids for the primary and secondary prevention of cardiovascular disease," *Cochrane Database Syst Rev.* 11, no. 11 (2018): CD003177, doi:10.1002/14651858.CD003177.pub4.

15. Monterey Bay Aquarium Foundation Seafood Watch, https://www.seafoodwatch.org.

16. C. D. Gardner, J. C. Hartle, R. D. Garrett, L. C. Offringa, and A. S. Wasserman, "Maximizing the intersection of human health and the health of the environment with regard to the amount and type of protein produced and consumed in the United States," *Nutr Rev.* 77, no. 4 (2019): 197–215, doi:10.1093/nutrit/nuy073.

17. B. Eisenhauer, S. Natoli, G. Liew, and V. M. Flood, "Lutein and Zeaxanthin-Food Sources, Bioavailability and Dietary Variety in Age-Related Macular Degeneration Protection," *Nutrients* 9, no. 2 (2017): 120, doi:10.3390/nu9020120.

18. National Institutes of Health Office of Dietary Supplements, "Choline Fact Sheet for Health Professionals," *National Institutes of Health*, Updated July 20, 2020, https://ods.od.nih.gov/factsheets/Choline-Health-Professional/.

19. G. A. Soliman, "Dietary Cholesterol and the Lack of Evidence in Cardiovascular Disease," *Nutrients* 10, no. 6 (2018): 780, doi:10.3390/nu10060780.

20. I. Berrazaga, V. Micard, M. Gueugneau, and S. Walrand, "The Role of the Anabolic Properties of Plant- versus Animal-Based Protein Sources in

Supporting Muscle Mass Maintenance: A Critical Review," *Nutrients* 11, no. 8 (2019): 1825, doi:10.3390/nu11081825.

21. J. Martinez and J. E. Lewi, "An unusual case of gynecomastia associated with soy product consumption," *Endocr Pract.* 14, no. 4 (2008): 415–18, doi:10.4158/EP.14.4.415.

22. N. Miyanaga, H. Akaza, S. Hinotsu, et al, "Prostate cancer chemoprevention study: an investigative randomized control study using purified isoflavones in men with rising prostate-specific antigen," *Cancer Sci.* 103, no. 1 (2012): 125–30, doi:10.1111/j.1349-7006.2011.02120.x.

23. M. Chen, Y. Rao, Y. Zheng, et al, "Association between soy isoflavone intake and breast cancer risk for pre- and post-menopausal women: a meta-analysis of epidemiological studies," *PLoS One* 9, no. 2 (2014): e89288, doi:10.1371/journal.pone.0089288.

24. S. M. Nachvak, S. Moradi, J. Anjom-Shoae, et al, "Soy, soy isoflavones, and protein intake in relation to mortality from all causes, cancers, and cardiovascular diseases: a systematic review and dose-response meta-analysis of prospective cohort studies," *J Acad Nutr Diet.* 119, no. 9 (2019): 1483–1500, e17, doi:10.1016/j.jand.2019.04.011.

25. M. Chen, Y. Rao, Y. Zheng, et al, "Association between soy isoflavone intake and breast cancer risk for pre- and post-menopausal women: a meta-analysis of epidemiological studies," *PLoS One* 9, no. 2 (2014): e89288, doi:10.1371/journal.pone.0089288.

26. M. Touillaud, A. Gelot, S. Mesrine, et al, "Use of dietary supplements containing soy isoflavones and breast cancer risk among women aged >50 y: a prospective study," *Am J Clin Nutr.* 109, no. 3 (2019): 597–605, doi:10.1093/ajcn/nqy313.

27. A. Mie, H. R. Andersen, S. Gunnarsson, et al, "Human health implications of organic food and organic agriculture: a comprehensive review," *Environ Health* 16, no. 1 (2017): 111, doi:10.1186/s12940-017-0315-4.

28. Carly Hyland, Asa Bradman, Roy Gerona, Sharyle Patton, Igor Zakharevich, Robert B. Gunier, and Kendra Klein, "Organic diet intervention significantly reduces urinary pesticide levels in U.S. children and adults," *Environmental Research* 171 (2019): 568–75, ISSN 0013–9351, doi:10.1016/j.envres.2019.01.024.

29. C. K. Winter and J. M. Katz, "Dietary exposure to pesticide residues from

commodities alleged to contain the highest contamination levels," *J Toxicol.* (2011): 589674, doi:10.1155/2011/589674.

30. Helen Thompson, "How did humans learn to digest milk?" *Genetic Literacy Project,* June 8, 2015, https://geneticliteracyproject.org/2015/06/08/how-did-humans-learn-to-digest-milk/.

31. C. M. Kerksick, S. Arent, B. J. Schoenfeld, et al, "International society of sports nutrition position stand: nutrient timing," *J Int Soc Sports Nutr.* 14 (2017): 33, doi:10.1186/s12970-017-0189-4.

32. A. A. Aragon and B. J. Schoenfeld, "Nutrient timing revisited: is there a post-exercise anabolic window?," *J Int Soc Sports Nutr.* 10, no. 1 (2013): 5, doi:10.1186/1550-2783-10-5.

chapter 7: make friends with fats

1. Ann F. La Berge, "How the Ideology of Low Fat Conquered America," *Journal of the History of Medicine and Allied Sciences* 63, no. 2 (April 2008): 139–77, doi:10.1093/jhmas/jrn001.

2. L. Tappy, "Thermic effect of food and sympathetic nervous system activity in humans," *Reprod Nutr Dev.* 36, no. 4 (1996): 391–97, doi:10.1051/rnd:19960405.

3. R. DuBroff, M. de Lorgeril, "Fat or fiction: the diet-heart hypothesis," *BMJ Evidence-Based Medicine,* first published online May 29, 2019, doi:10.1136/bmjebm-2019-111180.

4. V. W. Zhong, L. Van Horn, M. C. Cornelis, et al, "Associations of Dietary Cholesterol or Egg Consumption with Incident Cardiovascular Disease and Mortality," *JAMA* 321, no. 11 (2019): 1081–95, doi:10.1001/jama.2019.1572.

5. Mi Ah Han, Dena Zeraatkar, Gordon H. Guyatt, et al, "A Systematic Review and Meta-Analysis of Cohort Studies." *Annals of Internal Medicine* 171, no. 10 (2019): 711–20, doi:10.7326/M19-0699.

6. National Institutes of Health Office of Dietary Supplements, "Omega-3 Fatty Acids Fact Sheet for Health Professionals," *National Institutes of Health,* updated October 17, 2019, https://ods.od.nih.gov/factsheets/Omega3FattyAcids-HealthProfessional/.

7. J. J. DiNicolantonio and J. H. O'Keefe, "Importance of maintaining a low omega-6/omega-3 ratio for reducing inflammation," *Open Heart* 5 (2018): e000946, doi:10.1136/openhrt-2018-000946.

8. FDA, "FDA Approves New Qualified Health Claim for Oils High in Oleic Acid That Cut Risk of Coronary Heart Disease," *Today's Dietitian*, accessed July 19, 2020, https://www.todaysdietitian.com/news/exclusive1218.shtml.

9. Penny-Kris Etherton, Robert H. Eckel, Barbara V. Howard, et al, "Lyon Diet Heart Study," *Circulation* 103, no. 13 (2001): 1823–18253, doi:10 .1161/01.CIR.103.13.1823.

10. P. W. Siri-Tarino, Q. Sun Q, F. B. Hu, R. M. Krauss, "Meta-analysis of prospective cohort studies evaluating the association of saturated fat with cardiovascular disease," *Am J Clin Nutr*. 91, no. 3 (2010): 535–46, doi:10.3945/ajcn.2009.27725.

11. R. J. de Souza, A. Mente, A. Maroleanu, et al, "Intake of saturated and trans unsaturated fatty acids and risk of all cause mortality, cardiovascular disease, and type 2 diabetes: systematic review and meta-analysis of observational studies," *BMJ* 351 (2015): h3978, doi:10.1136/bmj.h3978.

12. Frank M. Sacks, Alice H. Lichtenstein, Jason H. Y. Wu, et al, "Dietary Fats and Cardiovascular Disease: A Presidential Advisory From the American Heart Association," *Circulation* 136, no. 3 (2017): e1–e23, doi:10.1161/ CIR.0000000000000510.

13. J. A. Nettleton, I. A. Brouwer, R. P. Mensink, C. Diekman, and G. Hornstra, "Fats in Foods: Current Evidence for Dietary Advice," *Ann Nutr Metab*. 72, no. 3 (2018): 248–54, doi:10.1159/000488006.

14. T. A. O'Sullivan, K. Hafekost, F. Mitrou, and D. Lawrence, "Food sources of saturated fat and the association with mortality: a meta-analysis," *Am J Public Health* 103, no. 9 (2013): e31–e42, doi:10.2105/ AJPH.2013.301492.

15. National Cancer Institute, "Identification of Top Food Sources of Various Dietary Components," *Epidemiology and Genomics Research Program*, updated November 30, 2019, https://epi.grants.cancer.gov/diet /foodsources.

16. M. D. White, A. A. Papamandjaris, and P. J. Jones, "Enhanced postprandial energy expenditure with medium-chain fatty acid feeding is attenuated after 14 d in premenopausal women," *Am J Clin Nutr*. 59, no. 5 (1999): 883–89, doi:10.1093/ajcn/69.5.883.

17. Renan da Silva Lima and Jane Mara Block, "Coconut oil: what do we really know about it so far?," *Food Quality and Safety* 3, no. 2 (May 2019): 61–72, doi:10.1093/fqsafe/fyz004.

18. Valentina Remig, Barry Franklin, Simeon Margolis, Georgia Kostas, Theresa Nece, and James C. Street, "Trans Fats in America: A Review of Their Use, Consumption, Health Implications, and Regulation," *Journal of the American Dietetic Association* 110, no. 4 (2010): 585–92, doi:10.1016/j.jada.2009.12.024.

19. C. Gayet-Boyer, F. Tenenhaus-Aziza, C. Prunet, et al, "Is there a linear relationship between the dose of ruminant trans-fatty acids and cardiovascular risk markers in healthy subjects: results from a systematic review and meta-regression of randomised clinical trials," *Br J Nutr.* 112, no.12 (2014): 1914–22, doi:10.1017/S0007114514002578.

20. J. Song, J. Park, J. Jung, et al, "Analysis of Trans Fat in Edible Oils with Cooking Process," *Toxicol Res.* 31, no. 3 (2015): 307–12, doi:10.5487/TR.2015.31.3.307.

21. G. A. Soliman, "Dietary Cholesterol and the Lack of Evidence in Cardiovascular Disease," *Nutrients* 10, no. 6 (2018): 780, doi:10.3390/nu10060780.

22. S. Chiu, P. T. Williams, and R. M. Krauss, "Effects of a very high saturated fat diet on LDL particles in adults with atherogenic dyslipidemia: A randomized controlled trial," *PLoS One* 12, no. 2 (2017): e0170664, doi:10.1371/journal.pone.0170664.

23. James J. DiNicolantonio and James H. O'Keefe, "Effects of dietary fats on blood lipids: a review of direct comparison trials." *Open Heart* 5, no. 2 (2018): e000871, doi:10.1136/openhrt-2018-000871.

chapter 8: rosé water all day

1. Heinz Valtin (with the technical assistance of Sheila A. Gorman), "'Drink at least eight glasses of water a day.' Really? Is there scientific evidence for '8 × 8'?," *American Journal of Physiology* 283, no. 5 (2002): R993–R1004, doi:10.1152/ajpregu.00365.2002.

2. Cleveland Clinic, "What the Color of Your Pee Says About You," *Cleveland Clinic*, October 31, 2013, https://health.clevelandclinic.org/what-the-color-of-your-urine-says-about-you-infographic.

3. Barry M. Popkin, Kristen E. D'Anci, and Irwin H. Rosenberg, "Water, hydration, and health," *Nutrition Reviews* 68, no. 8 (2010): 439–58, doi:10.1111/j.1753-4887.2010.00304.x.

4. James L. Lewis III, "Water and Sodium Balance," *Merck Manual,*

June 2020, https://www.merckmanuals.com/en-ca/professional/endocrine
-and-metabolic-disorders/fluid-metabolism/water-and-sodium-balance.

5. J. McNeil-Masuka and T. J. Boyer, "Insensible Fluid Loss," *StatPearls Publishing* (July 2019), https://www.ncbi.nlm.nih.gov/books/NBK544219.

6. Kamal Patel, "Caffeine," *Examine.com*, October 7, 2019, https://examine.com/supplements/caffeine/.

7. Diane C. Mitchell, Carol A. Knight, Jon Hockenberry, Robyn Teplansky, and Terryl J. Hartman, "Beverage caffeine intakes in the U.S.," *Food and Chemical Toxicology* 63 (2014): 136–42, doi:10.1016/j.fct.2013.10.042.

8. K. Yamagata, "Do Coffee Polyphenols Have a Preventive Action on Metabolic Syndrome Associated Endothelial Dysfunctions? An Assessment of the Current Evidence," *Antioxidants (Basel)* 7, no. 2 (2018): 26, doi:10.3390/antiox7020026.

9. Kamal Patel, "Caffeine."

10. U.S. Department of Agriculture, "Natural Peanut Butter," *FoodData Central*, updated November, 1, 2017, https://fdc.nal.usda.gov/fdc-app.html#/food-details/456107/nutrients.

11. U.S. Department of Agriculture, "Seeds, hemp seed, hulled," *FoodData Central*, April 1, 2019, https://fdc.nal.usda.gov/fdc-app.html#/food-details/170148/nutrients.

12. U.S. Department of Agriculture, "Raw Almonds," *FoodData Central*, updated July 14, 2017, https://fdc.nal.usda.gov/fdc-app.html#/food-details/487752/nutrients.

13. U.S. Department of Health & Human Services, "Guidelines for Alcohol," *Centers for Disease Control and Prevention*, accessed July 19, 2020, https://www.cdc.gov/alcohol/fact-sheets/moderate-drinking.htm.

14. Canadian Centre on Substance Use and Addiction, "Canada's Low-Risk Alcohol Drinking Guidelines," *Canadian Centre on Substance Use and Addiction*, 2018, https://www.ccsa.ca/sites/default/files/2019-09/2012-Canada-Low-Risk-Alcohol-Drinking-Guidelines-Brochure-en.pdf.

15. A. Y. Berman, R. A. Motechin, M. Y. Wiesenfeld, et al, "The therapeutic potential of resveratrol: a review of clinical trials," *npj Precision Oncology* 1, no. 35 (2017), doi:10.1038/s41698-017-0038-6.

16. S. Cains, C. Blomeley, M. Kollo, et al, "Agrp neuron activity is required for alcohol-induced overeating," *Nature Communications* 8, no. 14014 (2017), doi:10.1038/ncomms14014.

17. U.S. Department of Health and Human Services, "Alcohol Alert," *National Institute on Alcohol Abuse and Alcoholism* 46 (1999), https://pubs. niaaa.nih.gov/publications/aa46.htm.

18. Yin Cao, Walter C. Willett, Eric B. Rimm, L. StampferMeir, and Edward L. Giovannucci, "Light to moderate intake of alcohol, drinking patterns, and risk of cancer: results from two prospective US cohort studies," *BMJ* 351 (2015): h4238, doi:10.1136/bmj.h4238.

chapter 10: gut health

1. G. Vighi, F. Marcucci, L. Sensi L, G. Di Cara, and F. Frati, "Allergy and the gastrointestinal system," *Clin Exp Immunol*, 153 (2008): suppl 1, 3–6, doi:10.1111/j.1365-2249.2008.03713.x.

2. Hao Wang, Chuan-Xian Wei, Lu Min, and Ling-Yun Zhu, "Good or bad: gut bacteria in human health and diseases," *Biotechnology & Biotechnological Equipment* 32, no. 5 (2018): 1075–80, doi:10.1080/13102818 .2018.1481350.

3. V. K. Gupta, S. Paul, and C. Dutta, "Geography, Ethnicity or Subsistence-Specific Variations in Human Microbiome Composition and Diversity," *Frontiers Microbiology* 8 (2017): 1162, doi:10.3389/fmicb .2017.01162.

4. Bruno Senghor, Cheikh Sokhna, Raymond Ruimy, and Jean-Christophe Lagier, "Gut microbiota diversity according to dietary habits and geographical provenance," *Human Microbiome Journal* 7–8 (2018): 1–9, doi:10.1016/j.humic.2018.01.001.

5. B. A. Williams, L. J. Grant, M. J. Gidley, and D. Mikkelsen, "Gut Fermentation of Dietary Fibres: Physico-Chemistry of Plant Cell Walls and Implications for Health," *International Journal of Molecular Sciences* 18, no. 10 (2017): 2203, doi:10.3390/ijms18102203.

6. GMFH Editing Team, "Short-chain fatty acids," *Gut Microbiota for Health*, July 14, 2016, https://www.gutmicrobiotaforhealth.com/short-chain-fatty-acids/.

7. N. E. Diether and B. P. Willing, "Microbial Fermentation of Dietary Protein: An Important Factor in Diet–Microbe–Host Interaction," *Microorganisms* 7, no. 1 (2019): 19, doi:10.3390/microorganisms7010019.

8. A. K. DeGruttola, D. Low, A. Mizoguchi, and E. Mizoguchi, "Current Understanding of Dysbiosis in Disease in Human and Animal

Models," *Inflamm Bowel Dis.* 22, no. 5 (2016): 1137–50, doi:10.1097/MIB.0000000000000750.

9. Manon Oliero, "Understanding probiotics and their benefits: an ISAPP infographic," *Gut Microbiota for Health*, September 18, 2019, https://www.gutmicrobiotaforhealth.com/understanding-probiotics-and-their-benefits-an-isapp-infographic.

10. Monash University, "Prebiotic diet—FAQs," *Monash University*, updated February 2020, https://www.monash.edu/medicine/ccs/gastroenterology/prebiotic/faq.

11. M. J. Scourboutakos, B. Franco-Arellano, S. A. Murphy, S. Norsen, E. M. Comelli, M. R. L'Abbé, "Mismatch between Probiotic Benefits in Trials versus Food Products," *Nutrients* 9 (2017): 400, doi:10.3390/nu9040400.

12. Kristina Campbell, "Your guide to the difference between fermented foods and probiotics," *Gut Microbiota for Health*, July 26, 2017, https://www.gutmicrobiotaforhealth.com/guide-difference-fermented-foods-probiotics.

13. H. Zhang, C. Yeh, Z. Jin, et al, "Prospective study of probiotic supplementation results in immune stimulation and improvement of upper respiratory infection rate," *Synth Syst Biotechnol.* 3, no. 2 (2018): 113–20, doi:10.1016/j.synbio.2018.03.001.

14. Hanna Fjeldheim Dale, et al, "Probiotics in Irritable Bowel Syndrome: An Up-to-Date Systematic Review," *Nutrients* 11, no. 9 (2019): 2048, doi:10.3390/nu11092048.

15. C. L. Yang, J. Schnepp, and R. M. Tucker, "Increased Hunger, Food Cravings, Food Reward, and Portion Size Selection after Sleep Curtailment in Women Without Obesity," *Nutrients* 11, no. 3 (2019): 663, doi:10.3390/nu11030663.

16. R. Leproult and E. Van Cauter, "Role of sleep and sleep loss in hormonal release and metabolism," *Endocr Dev.* 17 (2010), 11–21, doi:10.1159/000262524.

17. SleepFoundation.org, "The Connection Between Sleep and Overeating," *SleepFoundation.org*, accessed July 19, 2020, https://www.sleepfoundation.org/articles/connection-between-sleep-and-overeating.

18. E. C. Hanlon, E. Tasali, R. Leproult, et al, "Sleep Restriction Enhances the Daily Rhythm of Circulating Levels of Endocannabinoid 2-Arachidonoylglycerol," *Sleep* 39, no. 3 (2016): 653–64, doi:10.5665/sleep.5546.

19. M. P. St.-Onge, A. Mikic, and C. E. Pietrolungo, "Effects of Diet on Sleep Quality," *Advances in Nutrition* 7, no. 5 (2016): 938–49, doi:10.3945/an.116.012336.

20. X. Meng, Y. Li, S. Li, et al, "Dietary Sources and Bioactivities of Melatonin," *Nutrients* 9, no. 4 (2017): 367, doi:10.3390/nu9040367.

21. W. R. Pigeon, M. Carr, C. Gorman, and M. L. Perlis, "Effects of a tart cherry juice beverage on the sleep of older adults with insomnia: a pilot study," *Journal of Medicinal Food* 13, no. 3 (2010): 579–83, doi:10.1089/jmf.2009.0096.

22. D. M. Richard, M. A. Dawes, C. W. Mathias, A. Acheson, N. Hill-Kapturczak, D. M. Dougherty, "*L*-Tryptophan: Basic Metabolic Functions, Behavioral Research and Therapeutic Indications," *International Journal of Tryptophan Research.* 2 (2009): 45–60, doi:10.4137/ijtr.s2129.

23. Emily Wax, RD, CNSC, "Magnesium in diet," *MedlinePlus*, updated February 2, 2019, https://medlineplus.gov/ency/article/002423.htm.

24. National Institutes of Health Office of Dietary Supplements, "Magnesium Fact Sheet for Health Professionals," *National Institutes of Health*, updated March 24, 2020, https://ods.od.nih.gov/factsheets/Magnesium-HealthProfessional/.

25. I. O. Ebrahim, C. M. Shapiro, A. J. Williams, and P. B. Fenwick, "Alcohol and Sleep I: Effects on Normal Sleep," *Alcohol Clin Exp Res.* 37 (2013): 539–49, doi:10.1111/acer.12006.

26. Michal Werbner, Yiftah Barsheshet, Nir Werbner, Mor Zigdon, Itamar Averbuch, et al, "Social-Stress-Responsive Microbiota Induces Stimulation of Self-Reactive Effector T Helper Cells," *mSystems* 4, no. 4 (2019): e00292-18, doi:10.1128/mSystems.00292-18.

27. J. P. Karl, A. M. Hatch, S. M. Arcidiacono, et al, "Effects of Psychological, Environmental and Physical Stressors on the Gut Microbiota," *Frontiers Microbiology* 9 (2018): 2013, doi:10.3389/fmicb.2018.02013.

28. J. R. Kelly, P. J. Kennedy, J. F. Cryan, T. G. Dinan, G. Clarke, and N. P. Hyland, "Breaking down the barriers: the gut microbiome, intestinal permeability and stress-related psychiatric disorders," *Frontiers of Cellular Neuroscience* 9 (2015): 392, doi:10.3389/fncel.2015.00392.

29. Cristina Rabasa and Suzanne Dickson, "Impact of stress on metabolism and energy balance," *Current Opinion in Behavioral Sciences* 9 (2016): 71–77, doi:9.10.1016/j.cobeha.2016.01.011.

30. A. J. Tomiyama, M. F. Dallman, and E. S. Epel, "Comfort food is comforting to those most stressed: evidence of the chronic stress response network in high stress women," *Psychoneuroendocrinology* 36, no. 10 (2011): 1513–19, doi:10.1016/j.psyneuen.2011.04.005.

31. R. R. Klatzkin, A. Baldassaro, and E. Hayden, "The impact of chronic stress on the predictors of acute stress-induced eating in women," *Appetite* 123 (2018): 343–51, doi:10.1016/j.appet.2018.01.007.

32. C. B. Ebbeling, J. F. Swain, H. A. Feldman, et al, "Effects of dietary composition on energy expenditure during weight-loss maintenance," *JAMA* 307, no. 24 (2012): 2627–34, doi:10.1001/jama.2012.6607.

33. K. Chandrasekhar, J. Kapoor, and S. Anishetty, "A prospective, randomized double-blind, placebo-controlled study of safety and efficacy of a high-concentration full-spectrum extract of ashwagandha root in reducing stress and anxiety in adults," *Indian J Psychol Med.* 34, no. 3 (2012): 255–62, doi:10.4103/0253-7176.106022.

34. Kamal Patel, "Ashwagandha," *Examine.com*, June 25, 2020, https://examine.com/supplements/ashwagandha/.

index

about the author

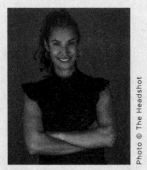

Photo © The Headshot

abby langer is a registered dietitian and owner of Abby Langer Nutrition. Her career has spanned over twenty years in various settings, from hospitals to private practice. She has made it her mission to debunk fad diets and nutrition myths and promote how to live your best life without dieting, both in her practice and in her writing. She has written for *Self* magazine, *Men's Health* magazine, and *Women's Health* magazine and has been featured as an expert in the *New York Times*, *The Cut*, and CBC Radio. She lives with her husband and two daughters in midtown Toronto.

abbylangernutrition.com
🐦 @langernutrition
📷 @langernutrition
📘 @abbylangernutrition